SERVE TO WIN

SERVE TO WIN

The 14-Day Gluten-Free Plan
for Physical and Mental Excellence

NOVAK DJOKOVIC

Foreword by William Davis, M.D.

Z ZINC INK   BALLANTINE BOOKS   NEW YORK

No book can replace the diagnostic expertise and medical advice of a trusted physician. Please be certain to consult with your doctor before making any decisions that affect your health, particularly if you suffer from any medical condition or have any symptom that may require treatment.

Published in the United States by Zinc Ink, an imprint of The Random House Publishing Group, a division of Random House LLC, New York, a Penguin Random House Company.

BALLANTINE and the HOUSE colophon are registered trademarks of Random House LLC.

ZINC INK is a trademark of David Zinczenko.

ISBN: 978-0-345-54898-6
eBook ISBN: 978-0-345-54899-3

Printed in the United States of America on acid-free paper

www.ballantinebooks.com

9 8 7 6 5 4 3 2 1

First Edition

To my family and friends,
my coaches and teammates,
who have worked so long and so hard
to make my dream a reality.

To Jelena Ristic, who means everything to me.

And to the people of Serbia.

We make a living by what we get, but we make a life
by what we give.

—Winston Churchill

CONTENTS

FOREWORD

P EAK HUMAN PERFORMANCE: That is what Novak Djokovic has accomplished in the world of tennis. Only a select few achieve this level in any field, and it takes a culmination of talent, courage, and determination—plus the removal of all impediments—to do so.

It's the aim of all human endeavors, from quantum physics to computer programming to tennis. For most of us, peak performance proves elusive, given the physical and emotional barriers placed in our way that impede achieving the true height of human body-and-mind potential.

Novak Djokovic has overcome overwhelming odds to achieve his exalted place in tennis history. He managed to obtain training experience in Serbia, a country in which tennis was virtually unknown. He maintained his demanding training discipline while his home city of Belgrade was under siege during the War of Kosovo, his family finding refuge in a bomb shelter for months on end. And yet, despite the hurdles he had to conquer, one thing nearly felled this champion. That thing was modern wheat.

Watching him in his 2010 Australian Open quarterfinal match against Jo-Wilfried Tsonga, you couldn't help but sense that something was impeding Djokovic's ability to stay at the top of his game: a mishit here, a millisecond of mistiming there, a wince with a tough return, and a medical timeout in the fourth set during which he appeared to be in visible abdominal discomfort. The result was defeat after several hours of struggle. His 2012 Australian Open final match against Rafael Nadal was an entirely different story: Djokovic was smooth, confident, and in control of the game—in a word, brilliant. How was this transformation possible? Simple. Djokovic removed the barriers to peak mental and physical performance by doing precisely the opposite of what conventional nutritional advice repeatedly tells us: He removed "healthy whole grains" from his diet.

As a result, he won three Grand Slam tournaments in 2011 (the Australian Open, Wimbledon, and the US Open), won an astonishing 50 out of 51 tournaments over 12 months, and earned the number one ranking for men's tennis in the world. His performance that year even astounded other top players, moving Rafael Nadal to declare that Djokovic's playing represented "the highest level of tennis that I ever saw."

How can removing a ubiquitous component of the human diet—wheat is found in virtually all processed foods—catapult an athlete's performance to new heights, allowing him to express his full mental and physical potential? That is precisely the question that I have devoted the last several years of my career to understanding: Why does modern wheat, the product of genetic manipulations by geneticists and agribusiness, potentially impair mental and physical performance, regardless of talent, ability, or drive?

I've seen it do so to staggering degrees. Modern wheat is capable of ruining digestive health, causing conditions ranging from acid reflux to ulcerative colitis and other forms of abdominal distress. It can trigger inflammation (common joint stiffness and pain) and autoimmune conditions (rheumatoid arthritis and Hashimoto's thyroiditis). It can unmask or worsen psychiatric conditions such as paranoia or schizophrenia and trigger behavioral outbursts and learning impairment in children with autistic spectrum disorder. It can cause weight gain, particularly in the abdomen, via its unique appetite-stimulating effect, making even athletes who train hours each day overweight. It can impair sports performance by provoking any of these and many other conditions, topped off with mind "fog," fatigue, and distortions of hormonal status, ultimately triggering a physical and emotional roller coaster that can strike anyone, anytime.

It struck Mr. Djokovic at that match against Tsonga in 2010—a match he knew he should have won.

As the father of a professional tennis player daughter, I can only begin to appreciate the extraordinary time and effort devoted to climbing to the top of the tennis world. Of all the hurdles one must face to achieve one's physical and mental peak, how can a simple nutritional misstep get in the way? Because eating wheat has always been the status quo, even at the lofty heights of the professional sports world, where it has the potential to cripple performance, cloud mental focus, and bring a champion to his knees.

It is a new age in sports performance. It is a new age in transforming ourselves in all spheres of life. It is a new age in rejecting the common advice to consume more "healthy whole grains." Mr. Djokovic's experience is perfectly consistent with what I have observed in hundreds of thousands, perhaps millions, of people who have followed the advice to cut all traces of modern wheat from their diet: staggering improvements in health and life performance.

I am thrilled that a noted public figure such as Novak Djokovic, someone admired and trusted by millions of tennis fans, has chosen to speak out on this issue and set a winning example of what can be achieved through exceptional commitment and hard work, coupled with genuine insight into maximizing performance through diet.

William Davis, M.D.
www.wheatbellyblog.com
Author of the #1 *New York Times* bestseller *Wheat Belly: Lose the Wheat, Lose the Weight, and Find Your Path Back to Health* and the *New York Times* bestseller *Wheat Belly Cookbook*

The Diet That Transformed Me

FROM THE BRINK OF FAILURE TO THE
CHAMPION OF THE WORLD—IN 18 MONTHS

UST AS I WAS REACHING for the top, I hit bottom. I was nineteen years old, an unknown kid from a war-torn country who had suddenly burst onto the professional scene. I was on a nine-match winning streak and poised to take a commanding lead in the final round of the 2006 Croatia Open. The stadium crowd was on my side; my team was cheering me on.

And yet I couldn't hear them. All I could hear was the roaring in my head. All I could feel was pain. Something was pinching my nose closed, bear-hugging my chest, pouring concrete into my legs.

I looked across the net at my opponent, Stanislas Wawrinka. I looked into the stands, where my mother sat. And then, suddenly, gravity sucked me backward onto the red clay court, and I was looking up at the open Croatian sky, my chest heaving. The Curse—the mysterious force that sapped my strength without warning—had closed in on me once more.

No matter how hard I inhaled, the air would not come.

My father, Srdjan, ran out onto the court and, with a doctor, lifted me up by my arms and sat me down in my courtside chair. I looked up at my mother, sobbing in the stands, and I knew. This tournament was over. And maybe my life's dream was over, too.

Most people don't decide what they want from life when they're six years old, but I had. Thirteen years earlier, sitting in the tiny living room over my parents' pizza parlor in the remote mountain town of Kopaonik in rural Serbia, I watched Pete Sampras win Wimbledon, and I knew: One day that would be me.

I'd never played tennis. No one I knew played tennis. In Serbia, tennis was as obscure a sport as, say, fencing. And the glamour of London was about as far as you could get from the desolate little resort town where my family lived. Yet at that very moment, I knew what I wanted more than anything: I wanted to lift the Wimbledon Cup over my head, hear the crowd cheer, and know I had become the number one player in the world.

My parents had bought me a little rainbow-colored racquet and some Wiffle balls when I was four, and I would entertain myself for hours, hitting the balls against the wall of the restaurant. But from the moment I saw Sampras that day,

I knew. And for the next thirteen years, I gave every day of my life to reaching my goal. My family, who made countless sacrifices; my friends who supported me from the beginning; my trainers and coaches and fans—they all came together to get me as close to my life's dream as possible.

But there was something about me that was broken, unhealthy, unfit. Some called it allergies, some called it asthma, some just called it being out of shape. But no matter what we called it, no one knew how to fix it.

It wasn't the first time I'd collapsed in a big tournament. A year earlier, ranked just 153rd in the world, I shocked 8th-seed Guillermo Coria by taking the first set of our match in my very first French Open appearance. But by the third set, my legs had turned to rock and I couldn't breathe, and finally I resigned. "Obviously, he was tired after a while," Coria remarked afterward. "When you're fit, you ought to be able to play a long match in hot weather."

Three months later, in the opening round of my first US Open, playing against Gael Monfils, I literally collapsed on the court. I lay on my back like a beached whale in the humid 80-degree heat, laboring for breath, waiting for a trainer. After four embarrassing time-outs, I managed to win that match, but I was booed off the court, and my lack of fitness was the talk of the tournament. "Maybe he ought to change some things," Monfils suggested.

I tried. In professional tennis today, the slightest change in your skill level, your physical conditioning, or your mindset makes all the difference. I practiced every morning and every afternoon, I lifted weights, I biked or ran for hours at a stretch every single day. It made no sense that I was unfit.

I changed trainers, looking for a new workout regimen. I changed coaches, thinking that something in my technique would free me from this curse. I had nasal surgery, hoping that would allow me to breathe more freely. Each change helped, a little; season by season, I grew a little stronger and fitter. In 2007, I became only the second player to beat both Roger Federer and Rafael Nadal since their ascent to the top of the game.

Yet every time I took a big step toward my dream, I felt as though a rope were around my torso, pulling me back. Professional tennis is one continuous, eleven-month-long season, and the key to consistency is being able to recover quickly from one match to the next. I'd win one tournament, then collapse unexpectedly in the next; win one epic match, then retire in the middle of the following round.

Maybe my problem wasn't physical, but mental: I took up meditation, then yoga, trying to calm my mind. My training became obsessive: For fourteen hours a day, every single day, I did nothing but focus on improving my mental and physical game. And in the process, I became one of the top ten tennis players in the world.

But I had a dream, and it wasn't to be *one of* the best. There were two men in the world who were the best—Federer and Nadal—and to them, I was nothing but an occasional annoyance, one who might quit at any moment when the going got tough. These guys were the elite; I was stuck somewhere in the second tier.

I won my first Grand Slam, the Australian Open, in January of 2008—a breakthrough. But a year later, against Andy Roddick, I once again had to retire from the tournament.

The defending champion, and I quit?! What was wrong with me? "Cramp, bird flu, anthrax, SARS, common cough and cold," Roddick said about me, making fun of the fact that I so often fell ill. Even Federer, who's so quiet and gentlemanly, dismissed me when talking to reporters: "I think he's a joke, you know, when it comes down to his injuries."

At the end of 2009, I even moved my training camp to Abu Dhabi, hoping that by practicing in the sizzling heat of the Persian Gulf, I'd be better prepared for the Australian Open in Melbourne. Maybe by acclimating myself better, I'd finally beat this thing.

And at first, it looked as though I'd finally figured it all out. By January 27, 2010, I'd made it to the quarterfinals of the Australian Open, handling my opposition easily along the way. Across the net in my quarterfinal match was Jo-Wilfried Tsonga, the tenth-ranked tennis player in the world. I was ranked number three. Two years earlier to the day, I'd beaten him on this very court on my way to winning my first Grand Slam tournament at age twenty-one. And on this day, I needed to be just as good. No, better.

Tsonga is two hundred pounds of pure muscle, one of the biggest and strongest players in the game, and his serve comes in at 140 miles an hour. When he puts his body weight into a return, the ball comes in "heavy," with a combination of speed and topspin that feels like it could knock the racquet right out of your hand. And yet he moves with great quickness around the court. On this day, in his neon yellow T-shirt, he looked as big as the sun, and just as relentless. He had taken the first set, 7–6, after a punishing tiebreaker that drove the crowd to their feet over and over again.

But by the second set, my obsessive preparation finally started to take over. I took that set, 7–6, and then I began to control him, running him back and forth along the baseline. The singles court is twenty-seven feet from side to side, and I could cover that distance as well as anyone.

I took the third set easily, 6–1. I had him.

And then it happened, again. With Tsonga up 1–0 in the fourth set, the invisible force attacked. I couldn't breathe. When he took the next game, something rose up in my throat; I pleaded with the chair umpire for a toilet break. I didn't want my opponent to see what I was about to do.

I raced into the locker room, burst into a stall, and fell to my knees. Gripping the side of the toilet bowl, my stomach in spasms, I felt as though I were vomiting up all of my strength.

When I walked back onto the court, I was a different player.

Tsonga knew my body was breaking down, and holding serve, he could run me back and forth across the court like a toy. I felt the crowd shift to his side, and his serve seemed faster, heavier—or maybe I was slower, weaker. It was as though I were playing against a giant. More than once, his shots left my feet stuck to the blue Plexicushion surface; I simply couldn't move them. He took the fourth set, 6–3.

By the start of the fifth set, it was clear to everyone in the park how this match would turn out. Serving 0–40, with Tsonga up 3–1, I hit the lowest point of my career. It was break point, in more ways than one.

I had to deliver a perfect serve, knock him off balance, regain some control. If there was one chance for me to battle back, I needed to make this serve the best of the hundreds of thousands I'd hit in my lifetime.

Bounce, bounce. I tossed the ball in the air. I tried to expand my torso to get full extension, but my entire chest felt tight. It was as though I were swinging Thor's hammer instead of a tennis racquet.

My body was broken.

Fault.

My mind was broken. Bounce, bounce. Serve.

Double-fault.

Game, Tsonga.

The end came quickly and mercifully, like an execution. After shaking hands at midcourt, he danced around the park, urging on the crowd, full of power and energy. I was drained. Seventeen years of practicing every single day, and yet I did not feel physically or mentally strong enough to be on the same court with the game's best.

I had the skills, the talent, the drive. I had the resources to try every kind of mental and physical training known to man, and access to the finest doctors in the world. What was really holding me back was something I'd never have suspected. I was training and practicing right.

But I was eating all wrong.

The Diet That Changed My Life

My professional low was that double-fault on January 27, 2010.

And yet, by July 2011—just eighteen months later—I was a different man. Eleven pounds lighter, stronger than ever, and healthier than I'd been since early childhood, I achieved my two life goals: to win Wimbledon and to be named the number one tennis player in the world. As I watched a last, desperate backhand from Rafael Nadal land long to give me the Wimbledon Cup, I saw myself as that six-year-old boy again, the one who came from nothing, innocently grasping at an impossible dream.

I fell to the ground. I threw my hands in the air. I crouched down, pulled some of the grass from the Wimbledon court, and ate it.

It tasted like sweat. My sweat. But I'd never tasted anything so sweet.

It wasn't a new training program that took me from being a very good player to the best player in the world in just eighteen months. It wasn't a new racquet, a new workout, a new coach, or even a new serve that helped me lose weight, find mental focus, and enjoy the best health of my life.

It was a new diet.

My life had changed because I had begun to eat the right foods for my body, in the way that my body demanded. In the first three months of my new diet, I dropped from 181 pounds to 172—my family and friends even began to worry that I was getting too skinny. But I felt fresher, more alert, and more energetic than I had in my life. I was faster, more flexible, and able to get to balls other players couldn't, yet I was still as strong as I'd ever been, and my mental focus was unshakable. I never felt tired or out of breath. My allergies abated; my asthma disappeared; my fears and doubts were replaced by confidence. I have not had a serious cold or flu in nearly three years.

Some sportswriters have called my 2011 season the greatest single year ever by a professional tennis player. I won ten titles, three Grand Slams, and forty-three consecutive matches. And the only thing I'd changed was what I was eating.

What amazed me the most was how simple these changes were to make, and how dramatic the results were. All I did was eliminate gluten—the protein found in wheat—for a few days, and my body instantly felt better. I was lighter, quicker, clearer in mind and spirit. After two weeks, I knew that my life had changed. I made a few more tweaks—cutting down on sugar, cutting out dairy—and I could tell the moment I woke up each morning that I was different than I had been, maybe since childhood. I sprang out of bed, ready to tear into the day ahead. And I realized that I had to share what I'd learned with others.

You do not have to be a professional athlete to make the simple nutritional adjustments outlined in this book, and you certainly don't have to be a tennis pro for them to improve your body, your health, and your outlook on life.

In fact, what I'm going to share with you isn't a diet in the strict sense of the word, because that implies that you're only going to eat exactly what I tell you to eat. That wouldn't make sense. Most diet programs assume the same plan works for everyone and that you "must" eat certain foods, whether you're a 27-year-old tennis player, a 35-year-old mother of two, or a 50-year-old executive vice president. That's silly. "Must" just isn't a good word. Your body is an entirely different machine from mine. Look at your fingertips: Your prints are unlike anyone else's in the world. This is proof that your *body* is different from anyone else's in the world. I don't want you to eat the best diet for *my* body. I'm going to show you how to find the best diet for your own unique self.

Simple Changes, Big Results

If you've been exercising to get fit, control your weight, and improve your energy, you've probably already figured something out: It's really hard.

I'm proof of that. For my entire career, I've played tennis for three to five hours almost every single day. I've competed in as many as ninety-seven professional tennis matches a year against the greatest players in the game. On days when I'm not playing, I still practice on the tennis court more than three hours, work out for another ninety minutes in the weight room, do a yoga or tai chi session, and, if I can, fit in some running, biking, or kayaking as well. And yet even with that training schedule, I was slow, easily winded, and a little overweight. My point is, if you think you're just going to exercise away your troubles, you'd better think again. I was training at least five hours a day, every single day, and I still wasn't fit enough. Was I carrying an extra nine pounds because I wasn't exercising enough?

No. I was heavy, slow, and tired because I was eating the way most of us eat. I ate like a Serb (and an American)—plenty of Italian food like pizza, pasta, and especially bread, as well as heavy meat dishes at least a couple of times a day. I snacked on candy bars and other sugary foods during matches, thinking they would help to keep my energy up, and figured my training schedule had earned me a handful off every cookie tray that passed by. But what I didn't realize was that eating this way causes a phenomenon called inflammation. Basically, your body reacts to food it doesn't like by sending you signals: stuffiness, achy joints, cramping bowels. Doctors have linked inflammation to everything from asthma to arthritis to heart disease and Alzheimer's.

Imagine you're hammering a nail into a plank of wood, and you accidentally hit your thumb. It hurts, right? Your thumb gets swollen and red and angry. That's inflammation. Now imagine that occurring inside your body, where you can't see it. That's what happens when we eat foods our bodies don't like. When I fell apart at the Australian Open, my body was telling me that I was beating myself up from the inside out.

I had to learn to listen to it.

Once I did, everything changed. And I don't mean just my tennis career. My entire life changed. You could call it magic—it sure felt like magic. But it was nothing more than trying different foods to find the ones that worked for me, and applying that knowledge to my daily diet.

Bottom line: I figured out which foods hurt me and which helped. It's not that difficult; I'll show you how (see chapter 4). Once you know the correct foods to eat, when to eat them, and how to maximize the benefits, you'll have a blueprint for remaking your body, and your life.

Here's how it works. You start by eliminating gluten from your diet for two weeks. (This is simpler than you think, as you'll read a little later on.) After that, you attack the excess sugar and dairy in your diet for two weeks, and see how you feel. (Here's a hint: You'll feel great.)

But changing what you eat isn't the end of it. You'll also learn to change the *way* you eat. You'll learn to sync your food with your body's needs, giving it exactly what it wants, when it wants it. And you'll learn how combining the right diet with proper stress-control techniques will improve the function of your body and your mind. You'll become more relaxed, more focused, more in control of your life.

In fact, what really inspired me to write this book is knowing that I can show you how to change not just your body but your whole experience of living—in just fourteen days. You will wake up more easily and feel more energetic, and you'll begin to see a difference in your appearance. Soon you'll be able to listen to your body, follow its cravings, and understand what it wants you to avoid.

Make no mistake: Your body will tell you different things than mine tells me. We're all different—we all have distinct fingerprints, remember? But the most important thing we can all do is listen.

On that day in January 2010, the tennis commentators thought they knew what was happening to me. "His asthma is acting up again," they said. And yet, as I double-faulted into the net, unable to breathe, I couldn't possibly know that I was experiencing something very different.

Since the age of thirteen I'd felt constantly stuffy, especially at night. I would wake up groggy, and it would take me a long time to get going. I was always tired. I felt bloated, even when I was training three times a day.

I had allergies, and on days when it was humid or the flowers were in full bloom, they would be worse. Yet what was happening to me didn't make sense. Asthma strikes as soon as you start to exercise; it doesn't come on three hours into a match. And my problem couldn't be conditioning. I worked as hard as anyone on the circuit. Yet in the big matches, against the best players, I would hold my own through the first few sets, then collapse.

But I wasn't a hypochondriac, or an asthmatic, or an athlete who just folded when the matches got tough. I was a man who was eating the wrong way. And my life was about to change. Who knew that the lowest point in my career would turn out to be the luckiest?

By sheer coincidence, a nutritionist from my home country of Serbia, Dr. Igor Cetojevic, happened to be flipping through the channels at his home in Cyprus when he came across my match in the Australian Open. He was no fan of tennis, but his wife liked the game, and she suggested they sit and watch. And they saw me collapse.

He knew it wasn't asthma. Something else was wrong with me. And the answer, he guessed, was food. More specifically, he guessed that my breathing issues were the result of an imbalance in my digestive system that was causing a buildup of toxins in my intestines. Which is a heck of a diagnosis to make from 8,700 miles away.

Dr. Cetojevic and my father had mutual friends—Serbia is a small country, after all—and six months after my disgrace in Australia, we arranged to meet during a Davis Cup match in Croatia. Dr. Cetojevic told me he thought food sensitivities were not only the cause of my physical breakdown but were playing a role in my mental state as well. He said that he could give me the guidelines that would help me create my own diet—the right diet for my body. He asked me about how I ate, how I slept, how I lived, and how I had grown up.

As a fellow Serb, Dr. Cetojevic could understand as well as anyone what my early life was like—what my family once had, what we'd lost, what we'd struggled so hard to overcome. A boy like me, growing up in Serbia, becoming a tennis champion? It was unlikely in even the best of circumstances.

And it became even more unlikely when the bombs started dropping.

SERVE TO WIN

CHAPTER 1

Backhands and Bomb Shelters

NOT EVERY TENNIS CHAMPION IS FORGED IN THE COUNTRY CLUBS OF THE WEALTHY

A LOUD BOOM SHOOK my bed, and the sound of shattering glass seemed to come from everywhere around me. I opened my eyes, but it did almost nothing to change my perspective. The entire apartment was inky darkness.

Another explosion and then, as though they'd also been shaken awake, the air raid sirens kicked in, and the loud black night became even louder with their screams.

It was as though we were living inside a snow globe and someone had hurled it to the floor.

"Nole! Nole!" My father cried out for me, using the nickname my family has called me since I was a toddler. "Your brothers!" My mother, leaping out of bed at the sound of the explosion, had slipped, fallen backward, and hit her head against the radiator. My father was trying to support her as she fought her way back to consciousness. But where were my brothers?

Marko was eight. Djordje was four. At eleven, I was the big brother, and I'd been holding myself responsible for their safety ever since NATO forces started bombing my hometown of Belgrade.

The bombings came as a surprise to us. In my youth, Serbia was still being ruled as a communist dictatorship, and very little information about what was really going on reached the general public. There had been rumors that NATO might attack, but no one knew for certain. Even as our government prepared for the bombings, we were kept in the dark.

Still, the rumors had spread, and like most families in Belgrade, we had a plan. Three hundred meters away, my aunt's family lived in a building with a bomb shelter. If we could make it there, we'd be safe.

Another soaring screech sounded overhead, and another explosion rocked our building. My mother had regained her senses, and we scrambled down the stairs and out into the unlit streets of Belgrade. The city was in total darkness, and with the air raid sirens blasting, we could barely see or hear. My parents raced down the pitch-black streets with my brothers in their arms, and I was right behind them—until I wasn't. My foot hit something, and I stumbled forward into the shadows.

I sprawled face-first onto the pavement, scraping my hands and knees. Lying on the cold concrete, I was suddenly alone.

"Mama! Papa!" I cried out, but they couldn't hear me. I

saw their forms growing smaller and dimmer, disappearing into the night.

And then it happened. From behind me, I heard something tearing open the sky, as though an enormous snow shovel were scraping ice off the clouds. Still sprawled on the ground, I turned and looked back at our home.

Rising up from over the roof of our building came the steel gray triangle of an F-117 bomber. I watched in horror as its great metal belly opened directly above me, and two laser-guided missiles dropped out of it, taking aim at my family, my friends, my neighborhood—everything I'd ever known.

What happened next would never leave me. Even today, loud sounds fill me with fear.

A Most Unlikely Meeting

Before the NATO bombing, my childhood was magic.

There is magic in all childhoods, but mine seemed especially blessed. I was blessed on that day when I saw Pete Sampras win Wimbledon and set my heart on following in his footsteps. But even more, I was blessed when, in the same year, the inconceivable happened: The government decided to build a tennis academy in the little mountain resort of Kopaonik, across the street from where my parents ran the Red Bull pizza parlor.

Kopaonik was a ski town, but it was where my family would summer to escape the heat of Belgrade. My family has always been athletic—my father was a competitive skier— and we loved football as well. But this flat green surface was something totally unfamiliar.

Like I said, no one I knew played tennis. No one I knew had even seen a tennis match in person. It simply wasn't a sport that Serbians paid attention to. So the fact that tennis courts were built anywhere was remarkable; but for them to be installed across the street from where I spent my summers? Some higher power was surely at work.

When classes began, I would stand at the fence, holding on to the chain link, watching the students play for hours. There was something about the rhythm and the order of the game that had me transfixed. Finally, after several days of watching me loiter, a woman walked up to me. Her name was Jelena Gencic, and she was the coach at the academy. She had also been a professional tennis player and had once coached Monica Seles.

"You know what this is? You want to play?" she asked me. "Come back tomorrow and we'll see."

The next day, I showed up with a tennis bag. Inside was everything a professional would need: racquet, water bottle, rolled-up towel, extra shirt, wristbands, and balls, all neatly folded into the case.

"Who packed this for you?" Jelena asked.

I was insulted. "I did," I told her, gathering up all my six-year-old pride.

Within a few days, Jelena began calling me her "golden child." She told my parents, "This is the greatest talent I have seen since Monica Seles." And she made my personal growth her mission.

Every day after school, I would ignore the other kids and their playdates and rush home to practice. Every day, I hit hundreds of forehands, hundreds of backhands, and hundreds of serves, until the basic movements of tennis became as natural to me as walking. My parents never pushed; my coach never nagged—no one had to force me to practice when I didn't want to. I always wanted to.

But Jelena didn't just teach me about sports. She became a partner with my family in my intellectual upbringing. The world around us was changing, and the communism we were born under was crumbling. My parents understood that the future would be a very different place, and that it was important for their children to become students of the world. Jelena had me listen to classical music and read poetry—Pushkin was her favorite—in order to calm and focus my mind. My family urged me to study languages, so I learned English and German and Italian in addition to my native Serbian. Tennis lessons and life lessons became one, and all I wanted to do was get on the court with Jelena and learn more about the sport, about myself, and about the world. And the whole time, I stayed focused on my dream. I would take different cups or bowls or pieces of plastic as my trophy, stand in front of the mirror, and say, "Nole is the champion! Nole is number one!"

I wasn't lacking in ambition. I wasn't lacking in opportunity. And according to Jelena, I wasn't lacking in talent. I was truly blessed.

And then came the war.

From Magic to Massacre

I watched as the twin rockets, birthed from the belly of the stealth bomber, tore across the sky above my head and sliced into a building just a few blocks away—a hospital. Instantly, it exploded, and the horizontal structure of the building made it look like a giant club sandwich stuffed with fire.

I remember the sandy, dusty, metallic smell in the air, and how the whole city seemed to glow like a ripe tangerine. Now I could see my parents in the distance, ducking and running, and I pushed myself up off the ground and tore down the street in the reddish gold light. We reached my aunt's building and barricaded ourselves inside the concrete shelter. There were other people from the building, around twenty families. All came down with their most valuable belongings, blankets, food, water, because nobody knew how long we would stay there. There were children crying. I didn't stop shivering for the rest of the night.

For seventy-eight straight nights, my family and I hid out in my aunt's bomb shelter. Every night at 8 P.M. there was a siren that announced the danger and everybody would leave their homes. The whole night we would listen to detonations, and when the airplanes flew low, there would be a horrible noise as if the sky were torn apart. The feeling of helplessness dominated our lives. There was nothing we could do but to sit and wait and hope and pray. Usually they would attack during the night, when the visibility was low. That's when you feel helpless the most; you don't see anything, but you know it's coming. You wait and wait, then you fall asleep, and then the horrible sound wakes you up.

But the war didn't stop me from pursuing tennis. During the days, I would meet Jelena somewhere in Belgrade to practice; she stuck by me and tried to help me live a normal life, even after her sister was fatally wounded when a wall collapsed on her. We'd go to the site of the most recent attacks, figuring that if they bombed one place yesterday, they probably wouldn't bomb it today. We played without nets, we played on broken concrete. My friend Ana Ivanovic even had to practice in an abandoned swimming pool. And when we dared, we snuck back to our local tennis club, Partizan.

Partizan was located near a military school. Of course, when NATO attacked us, they went first for the military bases to weaken the country's defense system—so Partizan wasn't the best place to spend one's time. But my love for tennis always prevailed, and despite the real threat, I felt safe there. Our tennis club became a getaway for me and most of my tennis peers. We practiced every day for four to five hours; we even played amateur tournaments during bombings, and it brought us so much joy that we could play tennis during wartime.

But even as we wondered whether we'd survive the war, my parents did everything they could to make life seem normal. My father was borrowing money everywhere he could to keep us living the same life we had always known. We were surrounded by death, but he did not want us to know that, did not want us to know how poor we were. And my mother was extremely strong, always finding a way to prepare food and let us lead our carefree childhood lives. We'd often have just a few hours of electricity a day, so she would have to be ready to cook as quickly as she could when the power came on, and get our meals finished before it went off again, making sure we had at least soup and sandwiches to eat.

Of course, my parents could do only so much to hide how much life had truly changed. Every morning there was a new crater, a new burned-out building, a new pile of rubble that had once been a home, a vehicle, a life. We held my twelfth birthday at Partizan. As my parents were singing "Happy Birthday," their voices were drowned out by the roar of bombers flying overhead.

Birth by Fire

We started the war living in fear. But somewhere during the course of the bombings, something changed—in me, in my family, in my people. We decided to stop being afraid. After so much death, so much destruction, we simply stopped hiding. Once you realize that you are truly powerless, a certain sense of freedom takes over. What will happen will happen, and there is nothing you can do to alter it.

In fact, my countrymen began to make fun of how ridiculous our situation was. NATO was bombing the bridges over the Danube, so sometimes you would see people gathered at the bridges with bull's-eyes painted on their shirts, daring the bombs to hit them. One friend of mine even dyed his hair to look like a bull's-eye.

These experiences became lessons. To truly accept your own powerlessness is incredibly liberating. Whenever I am extra nervous, not happy with something, or frustrated, whenever I feel like I am spoiled and I want more than I deserve, I try to refocus myself and remember growing up, remember how it was back then. That puts things back in perspective. I remember the things that I really value: family, fun, joy, happiness, love.

Love.

My biggest value in life is definitely love. It's what I always look out for and try to never take for granted. Because in a split second, life can turn around. As slow and as hard as your journey to the stars may be, no matter how many years it takes you to get there, you can lose it all in an instant. We have a saying in our country: Whenever nothing hurts, put a little stone in your shoe, and start walking. Always have that in your mind, because you have to be aware of the hardships others face. In the end, we are not created to be on this planet alone; we are created to learn from one another in unity and try to get this planet to be a better place.

Growing up in wartime taught me another crucial lesson: the importance of keeping an open mind and never ceasing to search for new ways of doing things. As a people, we were controlled by a government that kept information from us. The consequences of that continue to this day. Even though we have recovered from the war, we haven't recovered from the mindset that communism instilled: that there is only one way to think, one way to live, one way to eat. Tennis, and my studies with Jelena, opened my mind, and I was determined to keep it open. In the spring of 2013, as I was competing in the French Open, I received word that Jelena had passed away. But the lessons she taught me never left.

That's why, in 2010, when a skinny, gray-haired, mustachioed stranger approached me with a crazy story about how he'd seen me on TV and said he knew how to help me, I paid attention. Much of what Dr. Igor Cetojevic told me—about health, about life, and, most of all, about food—will strike you as truly unbelievable. But then again, so will the results.

CHAPTER 2

The Sweet Taste of Victory

A SIMPLE CHANGE IN HOW I ATE BROUGHT MY TWO LIFELONG DREAMS TO FRUITION

IT WAS JULY 3, 2011, and the sky above the All England Club was as colorless as our traditional Wimbledon whites. But despite the complete cloud cover, there was no rain in the forecast. The retractable roof would remain open for this, my first Wimbledon final. I jogged out onto the grass court, followed by my opponent, the defending champion, Rafael Nadal.

It had been eighteen months since my meltdown in Australia, and just a year since Dr. Cetojevic had introduced me to the idea that food intolerance might be the cause. And it was already clear to everyone in the tennis world that I had suddenly, seemingly inexplicably, become a different player.

The Association of Tennis Professionals (ATP) accords its rankings based on the previous twelve months' performance, awarding a certain number of points for reaching each stage of a tournament, points the player then has to defend when the same tournament comes around the following year. Since January of 2011, I had won fifty out of the fifty-one matches I'd played, and my success—including, at one point, forty-three straight matches without a loss—had been so dominant that the day before, when I beat Jo-Wilfried Tsonga to reach the Wimbledon finals, I was ensured of the number one ranking. My win made me the first man in seven and a half years to hold that position who wasn't named either Roger or Rafael. Just a year after changing my diet, my dream was coming true.

Maybe. Here I was, the number one ranked player in the world, on a record-setting win streak, having already beaten Nadal all four times we'd met so far this year. So as we strode out onto the Wimbledon court, it was obvious to everyone who the favorite would be to win this championship.

Him.

Yes, it was true.

Despite my ranking, Nadal—the defending champion, riding on a twenty-match win streak at the All England Club—was still the favorite. He'd won Wimbledon twice before. More important, he had beaten me in every Grand Slam match we'd ever had.

The experts all agreed. Before the match, John McEnroe declared that Nadal would win. So did Björn Borg. Pat Cash. Tim Henman. And pretty much everyone else in the know in professional tennis. I may have been the number one player statistically, but in everyone's mind, I was still that goofy kid from Serbia who melted down in the big tournaments when the going got tough. And the going is never tougher than when Rafa is on the other side of the net.

I would never truly be thought of as number one until I won Wimbledon.

A Gamble for the Win

Nadal is the strongest player on the circuit, and the most meticulous—a ball of nervous tics and superstitious rituals. In fact, I got him just a little upset a few years ago when I did an impersonation of him in front of the US Open crowd: Before he serves, he has to pull up his socks so they are exactly even with each other. Then he yanks his pants out in the back, and then bounces the ball into submission—twenty, thirty, fifty times even. All I had to do was grab the back of my pants and the whole stadium knew who I was pretending to be. Nadal also avoids touching the lines of the tennis court unless the ball is actually in play, always stepping over each line with his right foot, then his left.

But while he's calming himself with these rituals, he's also driving his opponents to distraction, which is not where you want to be when you're facing a player like him.

One reason is his forehand. The natural strength of most tennis players is their cross-court forehand, and their greatest power is when they drive the ball with a full swing, bringing the racquet across the body and the ball across the court to the opposite side. Nadal hits that forehand harder than anyone; it's been clocked at ninety-five miles an hour.

But that's not even the scary part. Nadal is left-handed, which complicates the equation. See, when two right-handed players battle, their cross-court forehands go to their opponent's forehand. As a lefty, Nadal is driving his massive, 95 mph forehand to his opponent's backhand. That means his strongest shot goes to most players' weakest.

At the coin toss, I stood nervously, while Rafa jogged in place like a boxer, part of his religious routine. Maybe he was keeping warm, maybe it was his superstitious nature, or maybe he was trying to intimidate me with his bouncing pecs. If I had pecs like that, I'd be bouncing around all the time, too.

My goal against Rafa was to not make the unforced errors, and to keep the ball moving quickly and consistently; in the past, it had been I who made the errors. But this time I had a plan to play very aggressively, and not give Nadal a chance to dictate. Typically, a big player like Nadal makes his opponent back up; the ball is coming so fast that the average player moves back to give himself an extra split-second to react. But my strategy was the opposite: I positioned myself right behind the baseline to cut down on the reaction time for us both. I was betting that my speed and agility would let me get to Nadal's best shots, and that by making the game quicker, I could prevent him from dictating its pace. If I could capture the energy of his shots, I could return them at the same speed, essentially using Nadal's strength against him.

It was a gamble, especially against that forehand. But while Nadal may have had a unique physical advantage, I had one of my own. Since losing the extra weight, I had become ridiculously flexible. Not many players, even at an elite level, can stretch their bodies to the point that I could, and the Wimbledon grass let me take particular advantage of that trait. One thing I had become known for was my ability to slide back and forth on the court—literally skidding from one side to the other and reaching extremely low to get to a return. That flexibility allowed me to cover more ground than the typical player. I didn't have to get as close to the ball as another player might—I could return it with power no matter how far I had to stretch.

I would need every millimeter of reach to win.

The Art of Discipline

What does it take to become the number one player in the world?

Every morning when I wake up, I drink a glass of water and do my stretching, maybe mixed with some yoga or tai chi, for twenty minutes. I eat a breakfast perfectly calibrated to feed my body for the day ahead—the same breakfast almost every day of my life. At about 8:30 I meet up with my coach and my physiotherapist, who will be with me every moment until just before I go to sleep, watching everything I eat and drink, and every movement I make. They are there with me every single day, all year long, whether it's May in Paris or August in New York or January in Australia.

I hit with a training partner for an hour and a half every morning, rehydrating with warm water. I sip a specially created sports drink my trainer mixes, carefully measuring the vitamins, minerals, and electrolytes depending on my daily needs. I stretch more, get a sports massage, and eat lunch—

avoiding sugar and protein and picking out only the carbo-hydrates that fit with my gluten-free, dairy-free diet.

Then it is time for my workout. I spend the next hour or so using weights or resistance bands—one set of high-rep, low-weight exercises for each of the different motions I must make, up to twenty different exercises. Midafternoon I have a protein drink made by my physio, one containing medical protein derived from peas. I stretch again, and then it is time for another training session, another ninety minutes of hitting the ball, looking for any slight hitch or deviation in my serves and returns. After that I stretch a fourth time, and maybe have another massage.

At this point, I have been training for nearly eight straight hours, and I now have a little time to attend to the business aspect of my career. Often that means a press conference or a brief charity event. Then I eat dinner—high protein, salad, no carbohydrates, no dessert. I might spend an hour or so reading, usually books on performance or mindful medita-tion, or writing in my diary. And finally I go to sleep.

That is what a "day off" looks like for me.

Unlike most other sports, there really is no "off-season" for tennis. Eleven months of the year, I have to be ready to play against the very best in the world—perhaps against the very best of all time.[1] To ensure my diet is the best possible, I get a blood test at least every six months to check my levels of

---

1. In 2012, ESPN asked Ivan Lendl—the number one tennis player in the world for most of the 1980s—how he thought he would fare against today's players. "My ass would get kicked so fast and so hard," he joked. But it's true—the precision level, skill level, and fitness level required to play top-ranked tennis today is entirely differ-ent from what it was even fifteen years ago. All sports evolve; tennis has just evolved faster than most.

vitamins and minerals and see whether my body is producing higher levels of antibodies, an indication I might be developing a sensitivity to a certain food. I sometimes use biofeedback machines to test my stress level. And I travel everywhere with my team: my manager, Edoardo Artaldi, who keeps me on schedule and sane; my physiotherapist, Miljan Amanovic, who monitors my physical well-being; my coach, Marian Vajda, and assistant coach Dusan Vemic, who make sure my technique never varies; and my girlfriend, Jelena Ristic, who cooks with me, trains with me, and keeps me on an even keel. Most of my inner circle is Serbian; they share the same terrible, war-torn past, and understand what it took for me to get to this point in life—and how impossible it once seemed.

When a tournament begins, I may have to play up to twenty hours of tennis over a two-week period, at the very top level of the sport. And that tournament may be in Melbourne or Miami or Monte Carlo, in California or Croatia or China, with perhaps only a few days off in between to get from one side of the globe to the other. Every moment of every day of my life is dedicated to staying in that number one position. It can be only discipline; there is no room for anything else.

How much discipline? In January 2012, I beat Nadal in the finals of the Australian Open. The match lasted five hours and fifty-three minutes—the longest match in Australian Open history, and the longest Grand Slam singles final in the Open Era. Many commentators have called that match the single greatest tennis match of all time.

After I won, I sat in the locker room in Melbourne. I

wanted one thing: to taste chocolate. I hadn't tasted it since the summer of 2010. Miljan brought me a candy bar. I broke off one square—one tiny square—and popped it into my mouth, let it melt on my tongue. That was all I would allow myself.

That is what it has taken to get to number one.

Raising the Cup

To win the 2011 Wimbledon Cup, I needed more than just discipline. I needed every ounce of training and skill I'd accumulated over the previous two decades. I was riddled with nerves—as was my whole team. Marian had to go for a forty-five-minute run before the match just to burn off some nervous energy.

I started the match with the serve. With every point I won, my team leapt to their feet and cheered—my family was with them, and Marko and Djordje in particular couldn't sit still. But with every point Nadal scored, his team remained as still and calm as a jury in its box. I may have been number one, but I was still the upstart.

Early in the first game, Nadal let me know the forehand was out in force, driving two identical bullets down the sideline to take a 15–30 lead. Fair warning: I needed to keep him moving wide so he couldn't get that impossible angle on me. By the middle of the first set, with me up 4–3, it was clear that my close-to-the-baseline strategy was working; I was getting Nadal's blistering forehands back to him so quickly I was catching him wrong-footed. Nadal wasn't used to players who could hold their own against him in long rallies, but I stayed toe-to-toe with him and took the first set, 6–4.

Now I could sense Rafa's confusion. The ball was moving lightning fast, yet I kept getting to shots that he was sure would be winners. By the time I took a 2–0 lead in the second set, I could feel the stadium crowd starting to shift its energy to me. Plenty among them had said my number one ranking was a statistical anomaly. Here, on the biggest stage in tennis, I could sense the whole world realizing that, at last, I had truly arrived. I took the second set easily, 6–1.

It is very rare for a singles player at this level to fight back down two sets to none, but Nadal had done it before, twice at Wimbledon. And there was the elephant on the court: Would Nole collapse? Would his "asthma" act up, his fitness levels fail, his mental concentration break? Nadal's serve, which I had handled up until now, suddenly seemed to scream in with even greater velocity, and his forehand was becoming more accurate. Serving 1–4, I double-faulted, and Nadal took the game and the serve. Fully in control now, it took him just four serves to close out the set, 6–1. I felt the crowd's loyalty shift back to Nadal. They had been rooting for the upstart, but Nadal was going to show them who the real champion was.

In the fourth set, the tide remained in Rafa's favor. I couldn't score a single point in the first game, and I was quickly down two games to none. Nadal was moving me around the court, but still, I was getting to his returns, sliding across the court like a skateboarder. I won the third game, slowing his momentum. Then I won the next game, taking a 4–3 lead, and the reality of what might be happening had begun to dawn on me. I took the next game, and suddenly, at 5–3, I was serving for the Wimbledon championship.

This was it. Everything I'd worked for was within my grasp, but Nadal wouldn't give it to me. He jumped out to a quick lead and then, tied 15–all, we battled through a fearsome rally, the crowd going wild as we drove each other to the edge again and again until Rafa flopped a forehand into the net. But he came back to tie it 30–all with another brutal forehand smash.

We could have battled toe-to-toe like this for a while, but something in me said that I needed to shake up this baseline game, to send Rafa a notice that the inevitable was upon him. I served, then surprised Nadal by racing to the net—serve and volley!—and slapped his return diagonally for a winner. He never expected it.

And he never expected this: championship point, Djokovic. I served, and we exchanged returns. Then it came: Nadal hit a backhand up the line, and before it even left his racquet, I knew it was long.

I fell backward onto the grass, and by the time my body hit the ground, I was six years old again. But this time, the trophy wasn't plastic. This time, it was real.

In the previous twenty-four hours, my two lifelong dreams had come true: to win Wimbledon and to be named the number one player in the world.

Not a bad couple of days at the office. But it wouldn't have been possible if I hadn't discovered how to eat.

CHAPTER 3

How Opening My Mind Changed My Body

ACHIEVE A NEW LEVEL OF SUCCESS BY SETTING ASIDE THE "RIGHT" WAY TO DO THINGS

"THIS IS A TEST that will help us see if your body is sensitive to certain foods," Dr. Cetojevic told me.

We were not in a hospital or lab or doctor's office. He was not drawing blood. There were no scanning devices or big, scary pieces of medical equipment. It was July 2010, at a tournament in Croatia, and Dr. Cetojevic was explaining to me that he thought he knew why I'd fallen apart so many times in the past, and how I could change my diet, my body, and my life for the better. Then he had me do something very strange.

He had me place my left hand on my belly and put my right arm straight out to the side.

"I want you to resist the pressure," he said as he pushed

down on my right arm. After a moment, he stopped. "This is what your body should feel like," he said.

Then, he gave me a slice of bread. Should I eat it?

"No." He laughed. "Hold it against your stomach, and put your right arm out again." Once more, he pushed down on my arm, explaining to me that this crude test would tell me whether or not I was sensitive to gluten, the protein in wheat, barley, rye, and other common bread grains.

This seemed like madness.

And yet, there was a noticeable difference. With the bread against my stomach, my arm struggled to resist Cetojevic's downward pressure. I was noticeably weaker.[2]

"This is a sign that your body is rejecting the wheat in the bread," he said. I had never heard the term "gluten intolerant," but I had just taken the first steps in learning how big a role food had played in my life, how much my traditional, wheat-based diet had been holding me back—and how much was in my power to change.

(By the way: I have found that this makes for an excellent party trick: Get someone in the room to assume the same stance—right arm out, left hand on belly—and test their strength. Then have them hold a cell phone against their stomach, and test again. The radiation from the cell phone causes the body to react negatively and weakens the arm's resistance, just as a food you're intolerant to will. It is an eye-opening revelation—and will make you think twice about carrying your cell phone in your pants pocket.)

Dr. Cetojevic then explained to me that there were other,

---

2. This test is called "kinesiological arm testing," and it's long been used as a diagnostic tool by natural healers. It is explored extensively in the book *Power Versus Force: The Hidden Determinants of Human Behavior,* by David R. Hawkins, M.D., Ph.D.

more scientific and more accurate ways of testing my sensitivities to certain foods. The best and most accurate is the ELISA test, which stands for enzyme-linked immunosorbent assay. It's a common blood test that's used for everything from drug testing to diagnosing malaria and HIV to testing for food allergies. (You'll read more about this in the next chapter.)

The ELISA test can teach us very specific things about our bodies' sensitivities to food. The most common sensitivities are to gluten, dairy, eggs, pork, soy, and nuts. Some of us have unusual sensitivities, or unexpected combinations of them; for example, my trainer, Miljan Amanovic, tested sensitive for pineapple and egg white. But once you know what you're sensitive to, you can make dramatic changes almost effortlessly. (By eliminating just these two foods, Miljan lost ten pounds in only a few weeks.)

When my blood test returned, the results were shocking: I was strongly intolerant to wheat and dairy, and had a mild sensitivity to tomatoes.

"If you want your body to respond the way you'd like it to, you will need to stop eating bread," Cetojevic said. "Stop eating cheese. Cut down on tomatoes."

"But, Doctor," I replied, "my parents own a pizza parlor!"

Breaking from Bread

I have learned a great deal about nutrition and the human body over the last three years, but my quest for information has been going on much longer than that. All of my life, I have been seeking knowledge, not just about tennis, but about the workings of the body and the mind.

Perhaps, in part, that's because knowledge was for so long withheld from me.

I was born on May 22, 1987, in a country that no longer exists: the communist country of Yugoslavia. When you live under communism for generations, as my family did, you learn to accept that there is only one way of doing things. The government and the society in which you live tell you that there is one way to dress, one way to worship, one way to exercise, one way to think. And of course, one way to eat.

Growing up in Serbia—the name my country returned to after the breakup of Yugoslavia—we ate in a very traditional way. Serbian foods are heavy foods: a lot of dairy, a lot of meat, and especially, a lot of bread. Bread is an important part of Serbian tradition, from the *cesnica* (a sweet bread) we traditionally break at Christmastime to breakfast foods like *kifli* (a crescent roll) and *pogacice* (a pastry). And when you are in wartime, bread is literally life; for many of us, there were times when it was all we had to eat. I know what it's like to have a family of five people with just ten euros to sustain us; you buy oil, sugar, flour—the cheapest stuff—and you make bread. One kilo of bread can stretch over three or four days. Even though my family never went truly hungry, for many, many months we lived having electricity and running water for only an hour or two a day. Bread sustained us.

Even when times were good, it was always there for us. Because Serbia is close to Italy, Italian cuisine is a strong influence, so when we weren't eating bread, we were eating pasta and, especially in my family, pizza. The Djokovic pizza parlor was our main source of income for most of my childhood, and, of course, it was home base for my earliest days at the tennis court across the street, where my life's journey began.

In other words, you may love wheat, rye, and other grains that go into making traditional breads, pastas, and pastries. But I promise, you don't love them more than I did.

It's quite possible that, because I relied on bread and dairy for so much of my young life, my body became increasingly sensitive to them. When we're young, our bodies can work through a lot of the challenges we present to them. That's a blessing, but it's also a curse. When you're young and strong, you can fight through the bad food, the stress, without necessarily getting sick or fatigued. But as we get older, and we stick to the same way of eating and living, we begin to experience problems. We need to make changes in the way we eat. The changes aren't that hard. And the rewards are astonishing.

New Food, New Life

The greatest gift that tennis has given me is not fortune and fame, or the opportunity to make a living doing what I love, or even the chance to inspire others, especially my Serbian countrymen. The great gift of tennis has been the opportunity to travel. It has allowed me to open my mind to what other cultures have to offer.

As I said, growing up under communism, you are not taught to be open minded. And there's a reason for this: If you are not open minded, then you can be easily manipulated. People at the top are very invested in making sure we do not question what we are told to believe. Whether it is a communist ruler or, for many of us, the rulers of the food and pharmaceutical industries, people at the top understand that most of us are led by fear.

You don't have to live under a dictatorship to be manipulated by fear. It's happening today, in every country in the world. We fear that we won't have enough—enough food, money, or security. We work and work and work, and fill our bodies with fast food and processed food, because we are afraid to slow down. Then our bodies rebel. And so we go to the doctor because we have problems with our stomach, with our head, with our back. We want a cure. We get pills to cure the symptoms, but they just push our problems under the rug.

This is the way that I lived. I needed to relearn not just how to eat but how to think about food.

As a young man, I was not taught about the different ways that other cultures view food. I didn't know about sushi, Chinese food, or the Eastern way of planning meals—things that today are a crucial part of my nutrition plan. There are many beautiful things about Serbian culture, but years of communist rule have left us with a lack of knowledge. What I've learned over the years of traveling and studying and researching and accepting is that there are differences between cultures, and you can take the best ideas from every culture and apply them to your life.

For example, one of the aspects of Chinese medicine that has helped guide me is the idea of the body clock—the notion that our bodies have a daily schedule, and that every organ in the body has a time when it is healing itself. According to Chinese tradition, each organ in our bodies is undergoing repair in roughly this order:

Lungs: 3–5 A.M. Some people believe that the reason many of us wake up coughing, even if we don't smoke and we take good care of our bodies, is that while we've been sleeping, our lungs have been clearing away debris. A poor diet makes the lungs' job that much harder.

Large intestine: 5–7 A.M. It's critical to drink water as soon as you wake up, since this is the time of day when the large intestine is working to move toxins out of your body. Water aids in that process.

Stomach: 7–9 A.M. This is the perfect time for breakfast, because your stomach is at its most efficient.

Spleen: 9–11 A.M.

Heart: 11 A.M.–1 P.M.

Small intestine: 1–3 P.M. If you're exposing your body to the wrong foods, this is the time of day when your body may send its strongest signals. If you experience indigestion, pain, or bloating in the early afternoon, it's a clear sign that your body is sensitive to one or more foods that you're feeding it, and you need to take a hard look at your diet.

Kidneys and bladder: 3–7 P.M. It's traditionally believed that feeling tired or sluggish during this period is another strong indication that you're eating too much of certain foods that your body is sensitive to. You're supposed to feel energetic in the midafternoon, not ready for a nap.

Pancreas: 7–9 P.M. The pancreas controls insulin, which processes sugar in the blood. A poor diet can trigger your body to crave sweets, especially during this time period.

Blood vessels and arteries: 9–11 P.M.

Liver and gallbladder: 11 P.M.–3 A.M. Sleep trouble can be another sign of food sensitivities. If you have difficulty falling asleep in this time frame, it may be because your liver is working too hard to rid the body of toxins.

The very idea of our organs operating on some sort of strict schedule seems absurd, as impossible as the idea of testing foods by holding them against your belly. But what matters is not whether you believe in or follow these particular approaches. What matters is that you are open minded. As I said at the beginning of this book, I am not prescribing anything; I'm not a doctor or a nutritionist. I am recommending only that you open your mind and give these various ideas a try, and that you listen to the signals your body is sending you. Try to step back and analyze from a distance what's happening inside your body. Be objective. Only you can know what foods are right for you; only you can translate what your body is trying to tell you.

Fourteen Days That Will Change Your Life

I said at age six that I wanted to be number one in the world, and by some miracle, my first coach, Jelena Gencic, took me seriously. She also believed that being the very best meant studying much more than just tennis. Listening to classical music, reading poetry, thinking intensely about the human condition—this was part of my early training, both at home with my parents and on the courts with Jelena. She not only opened my mind; she gave me the tools to keep it open. It was in part because of her that I continued through my early life to explore every kind of conditioning I could find, from tai chi to yoga, and to seek out new expertise. If I was going to be the best, I would leave no possibility unexplored.

And so when Dr. Cetojevic approached me with theories that to many of us might sound far-fetched, I was ready to listen. At that bizarre and shocking moment when my arm struggled under his pressure, I realized that the bread I was holding against my stomach was like kryptonite. I was ready to make some changes.

But the idea of giving up bread and other gluten-containing foods—foods that were so precious to me, so ingrained in my life, my family, and my culture—was scary. Then Dr. Cetojevic explained that I shouldn't pledge to give up bread forever. As the saying goes, forever is a very long time.

"Two weeks," he said. "You give it up for fourteen days, and then you call me."

It was hard at first. I craved the soft, chewy, comforting feel of bread. I craved crunchy pizza dough, sweet rolls, and all the foods that I learned contained wheat, things I had never suspected. (There's a whole list of sneaky sources of wheat on pages 41–43.) For the first week or so, I craved these foods, but I focused each day on staying disciplined, and fortunately, my family and friends—even though they thought I was crazy—supported me in my quest. But as the days rolled along, I began to feel different. I felt lighter, more energetic. The nighttime stuffiness I had lived with for fifteen years suddenly disappeared. By the end of the first week, I no longer wanted rolls and cookies and breads; it was as if a life-long craving had miraculously abated. Every day for the next week, I woke up feeling as though I'd had the best night's sleep of my life. I was beginning to believe.

And that's when Dr. Cetojevic suggested I eat a bagel.

This was the true test, he explained. Eliminate a food for fourteen days, then eat it and see what happens. And remarkably, the day after I introduced gluten back into my diet, I felt like I'd spent the night drinking whiskey! I was sluggish getting out of bed, just as I had been during my teenage years. I was dizzy. My stuffiness was back. I felt as though I'd woken up with a hangover.

"This is the proof," the doctor said. "This is what your body is giving you to show you it's intolerant."

And I pledged from that moment on that whatever my body told me, I'd listen.

CHAPTER 4

What's Slowing You Down?

THE FOODS THAT MAY BE SECRETLY SABOTAGING YOUR BODY AND MIND

BEING A PROFESSIONAL tennis player can be a very good life, or it can be very hard indeed.

Tennis is a very different sport from basketball or football or other team sports. It can be extremely lonely and very discouraging—more like being a musician than an athlete. There are nearly two thousand male players ranked by the Association of Tennis Professionals. Many of us, when we first start, are scrounging for dollars to support our profession, and to pay our way from one tournament to the next, because if you don't win, you don't get paid.

Once you have some degree of success, however, the living gets lavish. Traditionally, tennis, like golf, has been a sport that relies more on training, skill, and natural talent than on physical conditioning. At the peaks of their careers, people like Pete Sampras and Andre Agassi were fit, but they focused more on skill than on diet and fitness. Even today, among the top two hundred players in the world, many still eat whatever they want, don't think much about training other than the time they spend on the court, and enjoy their success—and all the indulgences it can buy—to the fullest. You can travel the world, make a million dollars a year, and have a very nice life, if you have the natural skills and the dedication to be a top tennis pro.

But once you get into the top forty or so, things change. Today's tennis players are so professional that fitness and nutrition are fundamental. The best players serve at speeds of more than 135 miles an hour, and forehands regularly top 80 miles an hour. Top seeds like Nadal, Federer, Tsonga, and Andy Murray are probably stronger, faster, and fitter than any tennis players who have ever strode the court before.

We're like precision instruments: If I am even the slightest bit off—if my body is reacting poorly to the foods I've eaten—I simply can't play at the level it takes to beat these guys.

More important, I can't be the friend, the brother, the son, the boyfriend, or the man I want to be, either. Eating the right foods gives me more than physical stamina; it gives me patience, focus, and a positive attitude. It allows me to be in the moment on the court, but also with the people I love. It lets me play at the highest level in every realm of life.

I bet you want to play at the highest level you can, too.

Then here is my suggestion: Begin by changing the foods you eat.

Food Sensitivity/Allergy Testing

Doctors use several methods to detect food sensitivities or allergies:

Medical history. A doctor will interview the patient about his or her diet to determine which foods may be causing a problem. This may also involve having the patient keep a detailed food diary of everything consumed over a certain period of time, including water.

Elimination. Based on medical history and diet, the doctor will have the patient remove suspect foods from the daily menu. Positive outcomes could mean the offending food has been identified.

Skin prick test. This is the common method for detecting many forms of allergies (environmental, pet, food, etc.). The doctor uses a small needle to inject an extract of the potential allergen under the skin of the patient's back or arm. Redness and swelling at the injection site indicates a "positive." The doctor will combine this result with your history of reactions to make a diagnosis.

The ELISA blood test. An ELISA (enzyme-linked immunosorbent assay) is a laboratory test used to detect substances in a patient's system. It's commonly used in testing for certain diseases (HIV or hepatitis B, for example), drugs, and, of

course, food allergies. In this case, the test indicates the level of food-specific antibodies (im-
munoglobulin E, or IgE) in the patient's blood.

Oral food challenge. This is the most accurate of
food allergy tests, but also the most involved
and time-consuming. The doctor feeds the patient possible offending foods and observes the
reaction (if any). The gold standard here is the
double-blind challenge, where neither the doctor nor the patient knows what's in each food
sample. This keeps both doctor and patient
from having bias.

If you suspect you may have food sensitivities or allergies and want to know for sure, ask
your doctor about testing.

That's what these next two chapters are all about: I'm
going to show you the foods that changed everything for me.
The foods I learned I had to avoid, and the foods I've adopted
into my optimum diet. You'll see how and what I eat. Even
though I don't recommend that you copy my diet down
to the last calorie, you can use this information to ask your
own questions and discover your own best fuels, your own
best methods, your own best results. And you can use my
experiences—and the scientific information in this book—to
make the changes you need.

All you have to do is try. And to me, the worst kind of
defeat is not failure per se. It's the decision not to try.

As for what you're about to read in this particular chapter, I'll say with a smile that I'm not a doctor or an expert in nutrition. Obviously, I've had some help on the research end of things, but here's how my food issues were explained to me by the people who helped me remake my diet, my body, and, ultimately, my life.

The Trouble with Gluten

Much more is known about gluten now than even a few years ago, and millions of people are healthier for it. Gluten is a protein found in grains like wheat, rye, and barley. It's the "glue" in wheat that makes bread doughy; without gluten, you wouldn't be able to toss a pizza crust in the air or roll out a pie dough. All wheat products have gluten, even healthy whole-grain products. This means that gluten is in the vast majority of foods we eat. Which ones, exactly? Well, here's a sampling:

- **BREAD, OF COURSE.** That includes English muffins, hamburger buns, flour tortillas, wraps, even unleavened bread like matzos.
- **ANY NOODLE OR PASTA MADE FROM WHEAT FLOUR.** That means whole-wheat pasta, "spinach" pasta, or any other pasta that includes wheat.
- **SWEET BAKED GOODS LIKE CAKE, MUFFINS, DOUGHNUTS, STICKY BUNS, AND PIECRUST.**
- **CRACKERS, PRETZELS, AND ANY SNACKS MADE WITH WHEAT FLOUR.**
- **BREAKFAST CEREALS,** even ones like corn flakes that

don't appear to contain wheat products (they do).
This includes sweet kids' stuff and "healthy" unsweetened adult varieties.

**ALCOHOLIC BEVERAGES LIKE BEER AND ANY OTHERS
BREWED FROM MALT** (some wine coolers are malt-
based). Certain vodkas are distilled from wheat.

Again, this is just a sampling. The fact is, people in developed nations eat a lot of carbohydrates, and a lot of grains in
particular. How often have you seen a loaf of bread or a box
of cereal advertising "whole grains" as a healthy choice?[3]

And those are just the foods that are recommended for a
healthy diet. Think about all the junk food we eat that's
loaded with wheat. Nowadays, wheat accounts for 20 percent
of all the calories we consume. Worse, today's wheat and
other grains are genetically modified in ways that seem to
upset our bodies even more. Scientists who research agricul-
tural genetics have found that much of the gluten in genetically modified wheat—which makes up almost 100 percent
of the wheat eaten on earth today—is structurally different
from anything that occurs in nature.[4]

Like I said earlier, if you don't have an open mind, you can
be easily manipulated into believing that there is only one

---

3. Of the twenty-six potential daily "servings" of each food detailed on the USDA's
old Food Pyramid, nearly half—eleven—were grains. These days, the USDA uses a
Food Plate to illustrate how much food people should eat, though not much has
changed: More than three-quarters of the plate is taken up by grains, fruits, and
vegetables. Keep the fruits and vegetables, but get rid of the grains!

4. The authoritative text on genetic modification in wheat is *Wheat Belly,* by William Davis, M.D. As Dr. Davis points out, "[O]ver the past fifty years, thousands of
new strains [of wheat] have made it to the human commercial food supply without a
single effort at safety testing."

way to do things—in this case, by food and drug manufacturers, who want us to eat as much grain as possible. Grains are cheap to produce and, in many cases, subsidized by governments, so it is in the food industry's best interests to keep feeding the idea that wheat, in particular, is healthy. More grains mean more health issues—obesity, diabetes, heart problems—which mean more medicines, which we take on top of our "healthy" whole grains. Food manufacturers get richer. Drug manufacturers get richer. And we get sicker.

It's sad. Bread was a lifeline for me and for my people during the bombing of Serbia. Now it's stealing the quality of our lives.

How Sensitive Is Your Body?

So . . . what exactly is the problem with gluten? There are several, actually.

Some peoples' bodies simply can't process gluten, and the resulting physical reactions can be severe. The most serious of these conditions is *celiac disease*, a full-blown allergy to gluten. With celiac, exposure to gluten can cause an inflammatory reaction in the small intestine—bloating, cramps, diarrhea, and fatigue. Skin rashes can also occur. The intestines also can't properly process vitamins and minerals in the presence of gluten, so celiac disease can lead to weight loss, anemia, osteoporosis, and malnutrition.

Celiac disease is a recognized medical condition and requires diagnosis and treatment from a doctor. You don't have to be born with celiac—you can develop it as you get older. Folks diagnosed with celiac must go on a gluten-free diet, and accidentally consuming even a small amount of gluten (it can hide in foods like soy sauce and in additives like caramel color) can lead to several days of horrible symptoms.

But many more people are like me: We have a sensitivity to the gluten in wheat products. As many as one in five people may have some degree of gluten intolerance, although that number is hard to pin down, because symptoms can range from mild to severe, and often strike several hours after we've eaten it. (And how many of us happen to suffer the impact of a gluten intolerance on international TV while a nutritionist in Crete is watching?) If 20 percent of our calories come from wheat, chances are that most of us go through our lives suffering constant gluten reactions—feeling bloated, tired, and weak—and simply assume that's what daily life is supposed to be like![5]

Eliminating gluten can lead to rapid weight loss, greater energy, and even the end of allergies and other immune-system reactions. But cutting gluten isn't just about feeling better physically. That day at the Australian Open, it wasn't only my body that was rebelling; it was my brain. I could not gain control of my focus or my emotions. And that is the secret gift of my new diet: I think and feel more clearly and positively. And I believe you will, too.[6]

5. A 2012 study in the *American Journal of Gastroenterology* looked at nearly three hundred patients over a ten-year period and found a definite nonceliac wheat sensitivity that broke down into two types: one with symptoms similar to celiac disease and one that looked more like a general food sensitivity, with complaints of fatigue and bloating. Either way, eliminating gluten was the way to go. SOURCE: *Am J Gastroenterol.* 2012 Dec;107(12):1898–906; Non-celiac wheat sensitivity diagnosed by double-blind placebo-controlled challenge: exploring a new clinical entity. Carroccio A. et al.

6. Research has linked celiac disease and gluten sensitivity to not just an intestinal reaction, but a nervous system reaction as well. A study review in *The Lancet*

Did Pizza Really Keep Me from Becoming #1?

Because my family owned a pizza parlor, the Red Bull, when I was growing up, I lived on pizza for years. It was so easy for me to just grab a slice (or three) when I was hungry. It seemed logical at the time, not just for convenience, but also from a training perspective. Pizza has tomatoes in the sauce, calcium and protein in the cheese, and carbs in the crust. And that was the problem: cheese and crust. I ate so much pizza for so many years, I suspect that I gave myself gluten and dairy sensitivities.

What a shame. My family makes *really good* pizza.

But there's a happy ending. Nowadays, having seen the success of my new diet, my family has opened a chain of gluten-free restaurants in Serbia. They're called, quite simply, Novak.

Where Gluten Hides

Someone like me, who relies on his body for a living, might recognize a food sensitivity to something like pork or strawberries much more easily, because we don't typically

---

Neurology found that gluten sensitivity could cause "neurological impairment" on various levels. This would explain how many patients complain of "brain fog" after consuming wheat products and report clearer thought, more focus, and more energy after eliminating gluten from the diet. SOURCE: *Lancet Neurol.* 2010 Mar;9(3):233–5. doi: 10.1016/S1474-4422(09)70357-6. Gluten sensitivity: an emerging issue behind neurological impairment? Volta U. et al.

eat ham or strawberries every day, and those foods don't often show up as hidden ingredients in other products. But wheat is sneakier. Even on days when I didn't eat bread or pasta, I didn't see any relief. And that's because one of the biggest problems for gluten-sensitive people is the sheer number of foods that contain wheat. It can take five or more hours for symptoms to occur, so if you avoid bread, cereal, and pasta all day, you might never connect the bloating and fatigue you experience at 7 P.M. to your lunch of Caesar salad and fried shrimp (you got it: croutons in the salad and breading on the shrimp). Yet it could very well be wheat sensitivity that's holding you back. The following foods may contain wheat products or come in contact with wheat products in the manufacturing phase. Some of them may surprise you . . .

MEAT MADE WITH FILLERS: This includes cold cuts, meat loaf, meatballs, hot dogs, sausages, poultry injected with broth, and imitation seafood.

CERTAIN EGG AND NUT PRODUCTS: Egg substitutes, dried egg products, dry roasted nuts, and peanut butter can be gluten culprits.

MARINADES AND SEASONINGS: Avoid products made with hydrolyzed vegetable protein and beware of marinades, miso, soy sauce, taco seasoning, and foods prepared with cream sauces or gravies. Also, check your ketchup label—some brands contain malt vinegar, which is made from barley.

CERTAIN MILK PRODUCTS: Steer clear of chocolate milk, milk shakes, frozen yogurt, flavored yogurt, cheese spreads, and cheese sauces. Definitely avoid malted milk and malted milk powders.

PROCESSED CHEESES: Skip processed cheeses and cottage or cream cheeses made with vegetable gum, food starch, or undisclosed preservatives.

ALTERNATIVE BREADS AND GRAINS: Watch out for bulgur, couscous, durum, einkorn, emmer, farina, graham flour, kamut, semolina, spelt, wheat bran, wheat germ, and barley products including malt, malt flavoring, and malt extract. (Buckwheat, however, is totally fine; despite its name, buckwheat is a grain.)

CERTAIN FRUIT AND VEGETABLE PREPARATIONS: French fries from fast-food restaurants (the same fryers are used to cook breaded foods), commercial salad dressings, fruit pie fillings, scalloped potatoes, creamed vegetables, and vegetables dipped in batters may contain gluten. Also, flour is used as a coating on some dried fruits.

VEGETARIAN PRODUCTS: Everything from veggie burgers to vegetarian chili and veggie sausages can contain gluten.

DESSERTS: Some ice creams (especially flavors containing cookie dough or brownies), frosting, candies and candy bars, marshmallows, cakes, cookies, and doughnuts are made with wheat, rye, or barley. Beware of puddings made with wheat flour, ice cream or sherbets that contain gluten stabilizers, ice cream cones, and licorice.

BEVERAGES: Avoid instant tea or coffee, coffee substitutes, chocolate drinks, and hot cocoa mixes. Also pass on beer, ale, lager, malted beverages, cereal beverages, and beverages that contain nondairy cream substitutes.

FRIED MEATS AND SEAFOOD: Skip anything with a crunchy coating, from fast-food fried chicken to the calamari served at a fancy steakhouse.

SURPRISING RANDOM SOURCES: Caramel coloring, communion wafers, some envelope glue, Play-Doh (not that you should be eating it anyway!), certain prescription meds, and cosmetics like lipstick and lip balm can be hidden sources of gluten.

I understand that this list of forbidden foods may make you think that avoiding gluten is impossible. But that's not true. In most cases, the foods on this list are processed, artificial foods. Real eggs, real meat, real fresh fruits and vegetables—they're all fine. And you don't have to swear off the other foods forever. *Give it two weeks.* That's what I suggest. Avoid gluten for fourteen days and see how you feel. Then, on day fifteen, have some bread and see what happens. Later in this chapter, you'll see the variety of gluten-free foods you *can* eat. I've managed to stay gluten-free and eat a healthy, balanced, satisfying diet that fuels a professional tennis career—and I probably have far less control over my schedule and where I eat than you do.

You *can* take control over your diet, and your life. All you have to do is try.

The Smart Sweet Life

One thing my friends have noticed is how much my moods and energy levels have evened out since changing my diet. I have always been an optimistic person, but over the last two years, even my low moments—losing a match, or suffering through my father's severe bout with respiratory problems—have simply been less low than might be expected. I'm no longer anxious, unfocused, or prone to smashing a racquet after a disappointment. (Although I reserve the right to do it once in a while—a little fire is always a good thing.)

Part of that evenness comes from eliminating the brain fog that gluten was causing. And part of it comes from the mental focus exercises I will talk about in later chapters. But a third element is that I keep my blood sugars at a steady level throughout the day, and I do it by eliminating foods that cause a spike in blood sugar, also known as glucose.

Eliminating foods that raise your blood sugar and cause spikes in insulin—the hormone that manages glucose—can improve your health in several ways. One, you stop having food highs and lows during your day that lead to cravings, bingeing, and "sugar crashes." Two, having stable blood sugar will discourage your body from storing fat—something it does when there's too much glucose for it to use. And three, it becomes much easier to eat nutrient-dense foods like vegetables and lean meats because you're no longer a slave to wild food cravings and desperate feelings of hunger. More on that last one in a moment.

Now, when you think of foods that spike your insulin, you generally think of sugary foods: candy, ice cream, honey, or cookies. And it's true, such foods raise your blood sugar and trigger an insulin response in your body. But you know what can raise your blood sugar even faster?

Wheat. Even whole wheat.

Here's how it works: You eat a high-carbohydrate food, either something loaded with sugar or something that transforms to blood sugar (glucose) as your body digests it. Your body wants to use the glucose as energy right away, but most people have no need for quick energy because they aren't trying to beat Roger Federer for a trophy in the next hour or so.

So now there's a problem: Your body has to get the sugar out of your blood somehow, because blood sugar is corrosive to your body's tissues. (That's why diabetics, who have poorly functioning blood-sugar management, can develop blindness, nerve damage, and heart disease.) So your body releases the hormone insulin, which triggers the cells in your liver and muscles, as well as fat cells throughout your body, to pull the glucose out of your blood and store it.

The higher your blood sugar, the more insulin you need, and the more fat storage you get. It's a vicious cycle that causes insulin receptors in your body to become less sensitive to insulin as time goes on, so your pancreas needs to produce more to get the job done. That's the beginning of diabetes. Meanwhile, your body is storing all this fat, much of it in and around your metabolic center: your vital organs, or viscera. Called visceral fat, this is active tissue that releases toxins and causes inflammation in the parts of your body most important for long-term health (or unhealth). It invades and inhibits the function of your liver and your heart.

What happens if you don't eat insulin-spiking foods?

Your blood sugar remains steady. You don't have the up-and-down cravings for more sugary foods. Your appetite loses its edge because the foods you're eating—high-protein, high-fiber, high-nutrition—keep you feeling fuller, longer. Your body doesn't rot itself with excess glucose, burn out its pancreas, and store visceral fat. And your brain isn't suffering the roller-coaster ride of energy highs and lows.

Your system is healthy and properly fueled. You feel better and can attack physical goals with more energy and drive, which makes all your training—physical and mental—more effective.

Wheat and the Glycemic Index

One way to track the insulin-spiking ability of foods is by using the glycemic index. Created more than thirty years ago, it is crucial for diabetics and incredibly helpful to anyone who wants to control their body's insulin response. The faster a food raises your blood sugar (and subsequent insulin response), the higher its score. The index runs from zero (no insulin response) up past 100 (russet potatoes hit 111). As you can guess, once you get up past 50 on the index, you're talking about sugary foods.

Here's the surprising part: A lot of foods that are promoted as "healthy" have a higher glycemic index than foods that would universally be regarded as unhealthy. Wheat products in particular boost your blood sugar faster than regular old table sugar.

Based on information published by the American Diabetes Association and Harvard Medical School, here is a comparison of the glycemic index of certain foods:

Wheat Products

Whole-wheat bread	71
Cream of Wheat, instant	74
Grape-Nuts cereal	75
Puffed wheat	80
Pretzels, oven baked	83
Pizza, plain baked dough, served with Parmesan cheese and tomato sauce (a Djokovic staple for years)	80

"Sugary" foods

Honey	61
Sucrose (table sugar)	65
Orange	40
Peach, canned in light syrup	40
Potato chips	51
Ice cream, regular	57
Coca-Cola	63
Snickers bar	51

As you can see, whole-wheat bread raises your blood sugar almost 50 percent faster than a Snickers bar! Why? The main reason is how the carbohydrates in wheat are digested.[7] Between gluten and blood sugar spikes, wheat is the mixed-doubles team from hell. And you're all alone on the other side of the net. Once you cut wheat out of your diet, the gluten side effects disappear, of course, but you also lose weight. I chalk that up to better digestion and better blood sugar control.

I avoid *all* insulin spikers, and that means not just wheat

---

7. The primary carbohydrate in wheat, amylopectin, is broken down by the body faster and more efficiently than other carbohydrates. While amylopectin occurs in other foods, the specific version that appears in wheat is actually broken down and converted into glucose more easily than even other varieties of amylopectin. In short, it's like an express train for glucose.

So . . . what will happen if you give up one or all of these foods?

Let's say you give eating gluten-free a shot for two weeks. What can you expect? Depending on how big a role wheat plays in your diet—and remember, the average person gets 20 percent of his or her calories from wheat—you may experience some withdrawal symptoms. You'll need to manage those for two weeks: Don't go to the mall and sniff the Cinnabons. You'll just torture yourself. Plan your meals a few days ahead so you don't get caught starving and grabbing a sandwich out of desperation.

Believe me: The rewards will come quickly, and the cravings will pass. For me, removing gluten was like lifting a heavy, wet wool blanket that had covered my entire body. I lost weight. I felt lighter and more explosive in my step. My mind was clearer. After two weeks, I didn't want to go back.

Sometimes you accidentally have some gluten, and that's when you really see that your body has started to refuse these foods. You might experience slowness, dizziness, a foggy start to the morning, all the symptoms of a hangover. This is how your body lets you know that it no longer wants—or needs—these foods.

Listen to your body.

but also sugars and sugary products such as chocolate and soft drinks. As a result, I have a very simple diet: vegetables, beans, white meat, fish, and fruit. Most of the food is natural and hasn't been processed. You'll find that once you eliminate wheat, and the sugar spikes that come from it, resisting other sugary foods will become much easier.

One more important note about sugar, especially as it applies to active people and athletes: As you'll see in the next chapter, I do have sugar in my diet. But it's a very specific form of sugar—fructose, a natural sugar found in fruit and honey. I'm also vigilant about how much I consume. My goal while I'm training or playing a tennis match is to maintain a steady blood sugar. I can't have blood sugar spikes in competition.

My suggestion to you is to cut out as much sugar from your diet as you can. It's very simple: The less sugar you consume, the less insulin you produce, and the less fat your body will want to store. If you're active and burning off stored energy, so much the better.

Again, why not give it two weeks and see how you feel?

The Dairy Factor

Although my ELISA test showed a sensitivity to both gluten and dairy, it was important to monitor each change to my diet individually. At Dr. Cetojevic's suggestion, I started by giving up wheat for two weeks. This was a life-changer for me. I felt so much lighter and stronger that I decided to take the next step: I cut dairy out of my diet as well.

Now I was really raising eyebrows: The pounds were coming off quickly, and my family started to worry. How would I keep up my energy? Didn't I need dairy for protein? And how could I turn my back on pizza?

I can recommend to everyone the benefits of a gluten-free diet—even if you're not sensitive to gluten, the insulin spikes caused by wheat are truly unhealthy. But it's also worth experimenting with dairy products, because so many of us are lactose intolerant.

Lactose intolerance is a common condition in which the digestive system can't break down lactose, a sugar in dairy foods. The symptoms are no fun: bloating, gas, intestinal cramps, and sometimes vomiting. If you eliminate gluten and insulin-spikers for two weeks and still experience some of these symptoms, try eliminating dairy as well—milk, cheese, and ice cream, for starters.

If you do leave dairy behind, be careful: One of the biggest issues for people who can't eat dairy is consuming enough calcium to fortify their body (bones in particular). I'm not a fan of supplements. I prefer whole foods and natural sources for my nutrients. Some good alternative sources of calcium are broccoli and fish like tuna and salmon, and that's where I get mine; I love those foods. Fortified milk substitutes like almond milk are also very high in calcium.

Some lactose-intolerant people can eat dairy that has gone through a fermentation process, which reduces the lactose in the food. Anything with "live culture" on the label counts. If that's you, be careful: Yogurt is a good example of a live-culture food, but many yogurts have so much sugar added they're practically as bad for you as candy bars. Read the label before you buy.

And that point is worth noting: Dairy, while a good source of protein, isn't necessarily a "low-carb" food. It doesn't rank up there with candy bars and Coca-Cola, but did you know that an eight-ounce glass of 1 percent milk has 102 calories, and half of them come from sugar?

Say that again: Half of the calories in a glass of 1 percent milk come from sugar.

"That sounds crazy. How do you figure?" you might ask. It figures like this: Nutritionists calculate the calories in a food based on the amount of protein, fat, and carbohydrate grams present. Each gram of protein contains 4 calories. The same is true of carbohydrates. A gram of fat, on the other hand, contains 9 calories. So if you look at the total grams of protein and carbohydrate and multiply that by 4, and the total grams of fat and multiply that by 9, you'll get the total number of calories in a serving. Based on this formula, you can look at any food label and figure out how many calories from sugar are in a serving of the food.

So let's look at that glass of 1 percent milk. Per the USDA nutrition label, it contains:

Protein: 8 grams. Multiply that by 4 and you have 32 calories from protein.
Fat: 2 grams. Multiply that by 9 and you have 18 calories from fat.
Carbohydrates: 13 grams (from sugar). Multiply that by 4 and you have 52 calories from sugar.
Total calories: 102

And half from sugar. I'm not saying you shouldn't eat dairy or drink milk. I'm saying *I* shouldn't. Which leads to the next section, and a concept that is essential to any good diet: moderation.

At first glance it seems like there's nothing left to eat. But in fact, there's a whole world of fresh, healthy, delicious food out there—some to be consumed in large quantities, others in smaller doses. Soon, you're going to find that you're eating better than ever—and truly enjoying what you eat.

The Foods That Fuel You

Everything in life is about balance and moderation: in food, in exercise, in work, in love, in sex, in everything. (Okay, maybe a little less moderation in sex, but you get my meaning.)

I heard an old saying once that there are "four white deaths" in food: white bread, white sugar, white salt, white fat. That's not exactly true—I've already shown that whole-wheat bread is just as bad as white bread, for example. But the best guideline, no matter what your body type, is to avoid these four as much as possible and, when you do indulge, eat them only in moderation.

Actually, I try to moderate all the foods I eat, even the good ones. And as you'll see in the next chapter, *how* and *when* you eat are just as important, in my mind, as *what* you eat. But I've found that wherever I go, I'm looking for the following foods:

Meat, fish, and eggs. These may be the most obvious choices once you cut out all the wheat and sugar. I like chicken, turkey, and all kinds of fish. I eat one of these at least once or twice a day. When you factor in all the different ways you can prepare meat and fish, you literally have dozens of possibilities to choose from. While I do eat red meat, I focus mostly on fish and poultry, to cut down on fat as much as possible.

Whatever kind of meat or fish you eat, make sure it's of the highest quality. For fish, choose wild, not farmed. For meats, choose grass-fed beef and free-range chicken. Too many studies have shown that better, more natural environments produce healthier, more nutritious animals and fish.

As for eggs, I don't eat them much, because I don't eat a lot of protein in the morning, as you'll see from my diet plan starting on page 73. But at the end of the day they make a very healthy, easy meal if you don't feel like cooking meat.

Low-carb vegetables. Vegetables are the primary natural source of virtually every nutrient a human can need: vitamins, minerals, fiber, antioxidants. But not all vegetables are created equal.

Some vegetables are very heavy in starch and carbohydrates—beets, potatoes, parsnips, and other root vegetables in particular, as well as squash and pumpkin. Since I try to eat the majority of my carbohydrates during the day, for maximum energy, I typically avoid these at dinner because that's when I focus on protein. But leafy and stalk vegetables, like salad greens, broccoli, cauliflower, green beans, and asparagus, are what I call "neutral." Because they aren't high in carbs, I eat them any time of day.

Fruit. I eat fruit, but in a controlled way so I don't overload myself with sugar. Still, if you're going to have sugar, the natural fructose in fruit is the better kind. Plus, fruit delivers nutrients. I especially love berries of all kinds, but in small servings.

Grains (gluten-free). I most often go with quinoa, buckwheat, brown rice, and oats. Quinoa and buckwheat make a tasty gluten-free pasta.

Nuts and seeds. Raw, not roasted, are best. These are the foods that help keep me fueled and full as my training day goes on. They deliver protein without weighing me down, as well as other good stuff like fiber and monounsaturated fats. I like almonds, walnuts, peanuts (which you can't eat raw, by the way), sunflower seeds, pumpkin seeds, Brazil nuts, and pistachios.

Healthy oils. I stick with olive oil, coconut oil, avocado oil, and flaxseed oil when possible.

Legumes. I love chickpeas (the main ingredient in hummus) and lentils. Black beans and kidney beans are also good—high in fiber and nutrients. Avoid canned varieties, which jack up the salt content into unhealthy territory.

Condiments. The key is to avoid sugar-laden condiments like ketchup and barbecue sauce. Mustard, horseradish, vinegar, hot sauces, and wasabi are all tasty. And don't forget salsa, especially homemade.

Herbs and spices. There are too many to name here. Use them to make meals taste so amazing you won't miss the bread basket on the table.

That's a glimpse of what I eat. But how I eat, and why, is a big part of my professional and personal excellence plan. I'll explain these aspects in the next chapter.

CHAPTER 5

Serve to Win

A BETTER WAY TO EAT FOR MENTAL AND PHYSICAL PERFORMANCE

FOOD IS INFORMATION.

If you can remember these three words, they will change the way you eat. Food is information that tells your body how to operate.

If you want to know my real diet secret, don't ask me what I eat. Ask me *how* I eat. Because I believe that what I put in my mouth is only half the story. The other half is how the food communicates with my body, and how my body communicates with the food. I want my body and my food to become one, as quickly and efficiently as possible, with no fuss and no side effects.

In my country, we have a saying: "Energy comes from

your mouth." Every food you ingest changes your body in some way. It speaks to your body, influences it, directs it. When you become aware of this communication, and learn to facilitate it for the results you want, you will see the best physical and mental outcomes.

Here is how you join the conversation.

What "Slow Food" Means to Me

We live in a fast-food culture, and fast food means fast eating. Is it a race? Will someone give me money if I finish first?

A few years ago, as part of my quest to understand food, I went to a restaurant in London called Dans le Noir. There are now several of these restaurants around the world, and they are unlike any others—not for the food, but for the atmosphere. Because Dans le Noir is partially staffed by people who are totally blind, and when you eat, you eat in complete darkness.

I don't mean that they turn out the lights and you dine by candlelight. I mean black curtains, leave your cell phone at the door, complete and total darkness. A waiter meets you in the anteroom, tells you the selections, and writes down your order. Then he takes you by the hand and guides you in to immersive darkness, leading you, blind and helpless, to your table. You eat without ever catching a glimpse of your food.

And the food tastes extraordinary. Your senses of taste and smell are heightened, and flavors explode in ways you never thought possible. You eat slowly, naturally, exploring the meal with your nose and taste buds. The experience solidified in my mind just how important it is to slow down and resist today's fast-food mentality.

And that leads me to rule number one: *Eat slowly and consciously.*

As an athlete, I have a fast metabolism. My body requires a lot of energy, especially when I'm in a match. For that reason, I want to digest food as efficiently as possible so I conserve as much energy as possible. You must remember science class: Digestion requires blood. I need that blood when I'm performing. If I can help my digestive system work better and faster, I'll be able to get back to physical activity sooner, with more power in that physical activity. (By the way, this is why I drink primarily room-temperature water, never ice water. Ice draws blood to the digestive system to heat it up to body temperature. That slows the digestive process.)

If I eat quickly? I get the same result that you'd get if you shoveled it in. My stomach doesn't have time to process the information it's getting because it comes in the form of a big data dump of food. If the stomach doesn't get the right information in the right time, digestion slows down. Your body won't signal to you that you're full. You might overeat. You also don't give your mouth the time it needs to do its thing—namely, allow the enzymes in your saliva to break down the food in your mouth so your stomach doesn't have to. Again, science class: Digestion begins in the mouth. As you chew, the food breaks down, and your stomach has time to prepare for the food.

If I eat quickly, I'll have big chunks of half-chewed food in my belly and my body will have to work harder and use more energy to break it down. Simply put, I won't give my body the clear signals it needs to become one with the food.

That may sound strange, but I'll say it again: Your body needs to become one with the food. That is exactly what the process of digestion is.

When I sit down to eat, I start by saying a short prayer. I don't speak to a specific God, or follow the tenets of a specific religion when I pray, and I don't pray out loud—it is simply a conversation that happens inside of me. When I do this, I remind myself that there are hundreds of millions, maybe billions, of people in the world today who are worried about food. Living through a war probably helped me understand that in a way I wouldn't have otherwise, but I never take food for granted. I remind myself that I must always see it as a blessing.

When I sit down to eat, I don't watch TV. I don't check e-mails, send texts, talk on the phone, or engage in heavy conversations. When I take a bite, I often put my fork down on the plate, and concentrate on chewing. As I chew, the process of digestion is already starting. The enzymes in my saliva mix with the food, so that when it hits my stomach it is a fully formed piece of "information." It is the same as if you gave someone directions to your house; the more details you give, the more easily the person can get there, and the less time she needs to spend figuring it out. I want my body not to have to figure anything out, because I know how much it means to my stomach and to my energy level for the next part of the day. That leads to my second rule.

Rule number two: *Give your body clear instructions.*

What do I want my body to do with the food I'm feeding it?

Our bodies use food for two primary purposes: first, for energy, to keep our legs moving, our hearts beating, our racquets swinging. Carbohydrates are the primary source of energy for our daily activities.

Second, for healing and repair: to undo the damage of the day, whether it's from a long workout or a long day at the office. Our bodies use protein (as well as other nutrients) to repair muscle, generate new blood cells, and replenish hormones.

But just as with an employee, you need to give your body a list of priorities: "First, I want you to do this. Then, I want you to do that." During the day, I want my body to be as energized as possible. I don't want it taking time from its busy schedule of training to do something else, even if that task is important. That's why the vast majority of the calories I eat in the first half of the day, up through lunch, are carbohydrates. When I eat carbs with very little protein, I am telling my body, "I need energy. Proceed as necessary." I feed my body gluten-free pasta, rice, oatmeal, and other gluten-free, carb-rich foods for daily energy.

At night, I don't need energy. I'm exhausted, and I want a good night's sleep. So at dinner, I will tell my body, "I need you to repair the mess I made. Please take this protein and do what needs to be done." This is when meat, chicken, and fish come heavily into play.

As I mentioned in chapter 4, fruits and vegetables are a big part of my diet, but they serve different needs at different times of the day. For breakfast, I eat plenty of berries and other sugary fruits, because I want that fast-burning energy. At lunch, I still eat fruit or vegetables of any kind. But at dinner, I'm looking to throttle back the carbs. So I'm still eating salads, leafy green vegetables, and other vegetables that are high in water content, but I'm avoiding most fruits (especially white fruits like apples and pears) and most root vegetables, which are high in carbohydrates.[8]

By eating this way, I'm making sure my body has the nutrients it needs, but I'm also ensuring that it has the information it needs. In the meal plan that follows, you'll see that this kind of eating is really quite simple.

Rule number three: *Stay positive.*

There is another reason why I won't watch TV while I eat: There's very little on TV that's positive.

I believe that food can deliver positive or negative energy depending on not just what food you eat, but also how you treat it. Before I tell you why, remember what I said: "Have an open mind." I once saw an *amazing* test that has to do with Eastern medicine. A researcher filled two glasses with water—the same kind of water and the same amounts. With one glass, he shared positive energy: love, joy, happiness, all the goodness of life. He nurtured it.

He gave the other glass all his negative energy: anger, fear, hostility. He swore at the glass.

Then he let both glasses of water sit unattended for several days.

The difference in the waters after a few days was immense. The water that had negative thoughts and influences directed

---

8. The fruits and vegetables highest in carbohydrates include potatoes (37g for a medium-sized russet potato), bananas (31g each), pears (27.5 g each), grapes (27g per cup), mangos (25g per cup), carrots (25g per cup), beets (17g per cup), and onions (15g per cup). And beware of dried fruits: Raisins have a whopping 115 grams of carbs per cup.

at it was tinted slightly green, as though algae were growing inside. The other glass was still bright and crystal clear.[9]

Sounds crazy, right? I know. But to me, that test is proof that every single thing in the world shares the same kind of energy—people, animals, the elements, everything.

Including food. *Especially* food.

I believe that if you are eating with some kind of fear or worry or anger, the taste of the food and the energy you get from it won't be as powerful. What you give is what you get. That's another reason I say a ritual prayer before I eat. I'm humble before the food. I appreciate it now more than ever. Because food and I didn't always get along so well.

Rule number four: *Go for quality, not quantity.*

In the sports world, athletes are always afraid that they don't have enough—enough fuel, enough hydration, enough nutrition. Like most athletes, I used to worry that I never had enough food. "What if I run out?" I'd constantly ask myself. "Will I have enough energy to sustain a whole day of practice?" I was always eating something more—I'd keep eating even when I felt full, and force myself to shove down an "energy bar" loaded with preservatives and sugars during practice. And subsequently I would put too much food in my stomach, too much information for it to process. When I cut out those high-calorie sources of nutrition, many people

9. A 2004 report in *The Journal of Alternative and Complementary Medicine* by Masaru Emoto, M.D., includes a photo essay of frozen water crystals from various sources, including photos of water after the water itself had been taken from glasses wrapped in paper with either positive or negative words typed on them. Positive energy seemed to result in clear, snowflake-like crystals, while the water exposed to negative energy had darker and ill-formed crystals. SOURCE: *The Journal of Alternative and Complementary Medicine.* 2004; 10(3): 19–21. Healing with Water. Emoto M.

around me doubted what I was doing. No whey-protein smoothies? No heaping plates of pasta? No pizza? They warned: You'll never have the strength and energy you need!

But I've learned that it is far more important to focus on the quality of what you're eating than on whether you're eating too little or too much.

And I'm not just talking about "healthy" foods. Many of us know what healthy food looks like. But there are degrees of healthy food. There is a difference between a fresh tomato and a processed, preserved sauce made from tomatoes. I try to eat foods that are organic, natural, and as unprocessed as possible. The energy you get from these foods is cleaner, and therefore the digestive process is faster. Think of the last time you were in a hotel, or a spa. There was probably a bowl of apples there—bright, shiny, perfect. Nobody really eats them; they could be there for days. Weeks. They never seem to go bad. When you think about that, it's disturbing. Too much of our food is sprayed with pesticides and antifungal agents, and we truly don't know what these chemicals do once they are inside our bodies. What *are* they telling our bodies to do, exactly? A lot of studies have concluded that one of the things they instruct our bodies to do is to gain weight.[10]

At the start, everything is organic, because we take it from the earth. But then we treat it with pesticides, antibiotics, or

10. Nine of the ten most common pesticides are known "endocrine disrupting chemicals," which have been linked over and over again to weight gain. Research at the University of California at Irvine has shown that when we are exposed to pesticides at an early age, these chemicals can actually trigger a genetic switch that predisposes our bodies to gain weight. *The New American Diet: How Secret "Obesogens" Are Making Us Fat,* by Stephen Perrine and Heather Hurlock, contains a lot of additional information on pesticides and other common chemicals that are linked to obesity.

specially engineered nutrients. Some are genetically modi-fied, like our wheat. I understand—it's a business. The grow-ers want to make the foods look bigger and better. They want to sell more of it. They focus on quantity instead of quality.

Organic food is more expensive, of course, and so are things like wild fish, grass-fed beef, and free-range chicken. To me, all of these products are well worth it. Not everyone has the money to spend on "special" food, but if you can, I say do it. A surefire way to make organic options more af-fordable is to do what I do: cook. Even though I'm in a differ-ent city (and sometimes a different country!) every two weeks, I cook almost all of my meals myself.

I try to find a hotel with a kitchen in the room so we can prepare our own meals. My family often travels with me, and my girlfriend or mother makes sure the refrigerator and shelves are stocked with healthy foods. This way, I can con-trol the ingredients, portions, and timing. I also keep a lot of high-quality food around for the rest of my needs: fresh fruit in my fridge, nuts, seeds, coconut water, coconut oil, avo-cado, fresh fish . . . but more on these, and the dishes I pre-pare with them, a little later.

You Are What You Eat

My dietary changes—and the success I've had since I made them—have gotten a lot of publicity. When I credited food with my newfound success, people started paying attention, and experimenting. Now, when I'm playing a tournament, I'll go to the food service tent, and when the cooks see me coming, they put my gluten-free pasta on the stove. A few years ago I was the only guy eating it. Now I see a lot of other tennis players eating gluten-free pasta. I don't know if it's because of me, because of their own gluten intolerance, or just because they realize a gluten-free diet helps them to digest better (as I said earlier, gluten itself is like a glue; food that contains gluten sticks together and takes more time to digest than gluten-free food). But one thing's for sure: When I first started eating gluten-free pasta, I didn't see a single other player having it. Now I do—men *and* women.

Word gets around so easily nowadays. I think awareness is spreading, not just for a gluten-free diet, but for healthy food and better nutrition in general. More so now than ever before, people know what is good for them and what isn't. People realize that processed, fast food isn't working, that the "convenience" of bad food makes their lives more stressful, not less.

But there is still a disconnect. I see it, and I bet you feel it. Knowing and doing are two different things. People know what they should eat, yet they still make the unhealthy choice.

This is why it is so important to see food as information. Ask yourself: *How do I feel when I eat something unhealthy?* Not immediately, when you still have the sugar/salt/fat taste in your mouth. But afterward. When you eat bad food, your body knows it. Your body sends a signal that screams, "This food is lousy and you're going to pay for it!" Some of those signals? You feel lethargic, or "blah," or you have indigestion. Maybe your head hurts, or you feel foggy.

If you have an unhealthy diet over the long term, your body sends more serious signals. You gain weight. Your chances of being diagnosed with diabetes, cancer, and heart disease go up. This, too, is your body talking to you. If you don't like the way you look and feel, this is information: Your body is telling you to change, or there are going to be problems.

Now ask yourself: *How do I feel when I eat something that's good for me?* For me, it's simple: I feel great. That's what I've learned, and it makes my food choices easy.

"So . . . how much do you eat?"

I get that question a lot. It's a good question. This goes back to my earlier point about everyone being unique. Chances are your nutritional needs are very different from mine. But one thing is true for everyone: If you eat too much, you're going to feel lousy.

Like most professional athletes, I used to worry about consuming enough energy. But trying to make sure I ate "enough" was sapping me. I'd feel it as soon as I picked up a racquet; I would not be dynamic, not fresh enough on the court, because I didn't digest my food in time. I'd bombarded my stomach with too much information.

For regular non-athletes out there, the fear is probably the opposite: *Am I eating too much?* As a result, there's a lot of portion measuring, calorie counting, and fussing over food.

Now, I'm a professional athlete. If I wanted, I could hire someone to manage my meals and count my calories for me. But no one can be a better expert on my nutritional needs than me, just as no one understands your nutritional needs better than you.

Eating slowly has helped me learn exactly how much I need to eat. That may sound very vague: "I go by feel." But it makes sense, and I'll bet you do it a bit even now yourself. Don't you have times during the day when you feel like you need fuel? Don't you know immediately when you've eaten too much? Or when you've filled up on lousy fuel? Sure you do. If you paid just a little more attention to those feelings, if you ate more slowly, and focused on your food, you'd get a real "sixth sense" for how much you need.

So when you hear stories of elite athletes bragging about the massive amounts of calories they eat while training, well, that works for them. But I have no idea how many calories I eat. And I bet all you could offer is a "best guess" about your own consumption. I'd much rather know my body and respect the fuel I put in it.

A Day on My Diet

Now I'll take you through an average day of eating. I will say this up front: This isn't a cut-and-dried plan. Every example I give here is a variable; some days I'll follow it, some days I won't. Again, it's about how I listen to and understand my body. My hope is that you'll get two things from this food log: one, a sense of how I remain constantly mindful of my food intake based on how I feel, and two, a *huge* number of ideas to experiment with yourself.

Back in chapter 3, you might remember, I mentioned a theory from Chinese medicine that says certain body parts prefer certain foods at certain times. I like this theory and try to adhere to it. But even I have trouble with it sometimes.

I'm always traveling for tennis, always crossing time zones, always adjusting to new places and new cultures. I keep this theory in the back of my mind and do my best.

What I am religious about, however, are the four rules described earlier:

Eat slowly and consciously.
Give your body clear instructions.
Stay positive.
Go for quality, not quantity.

Here's how they play out in my diet.

Good morning, honey

Most of us have morning rituals, but mine is probably stricter than most.

The first thing I do out of bed is to drink a tall glass of room-temperature water. I've just gone eight hours without drinking anything, and my body needs hydration in order to start functioning at its peak. Water is a critical part of the body's repair process. When you're dehydrated, you're short-changing that aspect of your bodily maintenance.

As I said earlier, I avoid ice water, for a reason. My schedule is one of constant training and practice. On most days I'll start with a series of stretches or yoga moves (you'll learn more about that in chapter 7). Any kind of exercise, even just stretching, requires good blood flow to the muscles. When you drink ice water, the body needs to send additional blood to the digestive system in order to heat the water to 98.6 degrees. There's some benefit to this process—heating the cold water burns a few additional calories. But it also slows digestion and diverts blood away from where I want it—in my muscles. So in the morning, and throughout the day, I drink primarily warm water.

(If you've read a lot about diet, you've probably heard that slow digestion is good—you want things to sit in your stomach and keep you from getting hungry. That might be a good idea if you're going to sit down and watch a four-hour tennis match. It's not a good idea if you're going to play one. And slow digestion means you're going to feel sluggish and not particularly eager to move, which means less exercise and more bloating and fatigue. So don't be too eager to sign up for a diet plan that "keeps you feeling full.")

The second thing I do might really surprise you: I eat two spoonfuls of honey. Every day. I try to get manuka honey, which comes from New Zealand. It is a dark honey made by bees that feed on the manuka tree (or tea tree), and has been shown to have even greater antibacterial properties than regular honey.

I know what you're thinking: Honey is sugar. Well, yes, it is. But your body needs sugar. In particular, it needs fructose, the sugar found in fruits, some vegetables, and especially honey. What it doesn't need is processed sucrose, the stuff in chocolate, soda, or most energy drinks that gives you an instant sugar shot in the body, where you feel like, "Wow!"

I don't like "wow." "Wow" is no good. If you have "wow" now, that means in thirty minutes you're going to have "woe." The bad sugar makes your blood sugar go up and down, up and down. You can't perform as an athlete that way.

Good sugars, like the natural sugars you find in fruit and honey (fructose), aren't as wild on the glycemic index. In fact, as you read in chapter 4, honey will actually cause less of an insulin spike than the whole-wheat toast that most "health-conscious" people eat.

After a little stretching or some light calisthenics, I'm ready for breakfast. Most days I have what I call the Power Bowl, a normal-sized bowl I fill with a mixture of:

Gluten-free muesli or oatmeal
A handful of mixed nuts—almonds, walnuts, peanuts
Some sunflower or pumpkin seeds
Fruits on the side, or sliced up in the bowl, like banana
    and all kinds of berries
A small scoop of coconut oil (I like it for electrolytes and
    minerals)
Rice milk, almond milk, or coconut water

As you can see, you can play around with the different ingredients and amounts. One bowl of these ingredients is generally enough for me. If I think that I will need something more—I rarely do—then I wait about twenty minutes and have a little gluten-free toasted bread, tuna fish, and some avocado. I love avocado; it's one of my favorites.

There is a specific reason I wait twenty minutes before I eat any heavy protein after a "normal" meal like this. As you might guess by now, it has to do with digestion and eating slowly. Your stomach digests carbohydrates and proteins differently. If you are digesting meat proteins and carbohydrates at the same time, the process of digestion is automatically slower, and you are making your stomach's life more difficult because you are making it use more energy. So I try to give my stomach time to adjust. It's like sending my stomach carbohydrate signals first, then heavy protein signals later.

Remember: Food is information.

As My Day Goes On . . .

For me, a typical lunch is gluten-free pasta with vegetables. The pasta is made from quinoa or buckwheat. As for the vegetables, the selection is vast. Arugula, roasted peppers, fresh tomatoes, sometimes cucumber, a lot of broccoli, a lot of cauliflower, green beans, carrots. I combine the vegetables with the pasta and some olive oil and a bit of salt. Mixing and matching works well for me. What I don't eat are heavy sauces like tomato sauce. Tomato sauces—even the kind your mom makes "from scratch" at home—typically start with canned ingredients, and that means additives. In addition, heavy sauces slow down digestion.

(I should say that on match days when I know I'll have to practice around noon and play a match around three, I have a heavy protein with my lunch, as a foundation for the match. But in general, pasta is all I need.)

During an average day, I need some fuel to keep me going through training and practice. Here's what I do, though what I need at an exact time varies widely.

During practice, I go through two bottles of an energy drink containing fructose extract. It's not too heavy in the stomach, but allows me to replenish. The ingredients I look for in a drink are electrolytes, magnesium, calcium, zinc, selenium, and vitamin C. The magnesium and calcium help with heart and muscle function and prevent cramps. If it's a humid day, I also have a hydration drink with electrolytes because I lose a lot of liquids.

Hydration is a big thing throughout the day, of course. No matter what I'm doing, I always try to have water with me. I've experienced dehydration before, and the signals for me are intense thirst, dizziness, a lack of energy and power, and sometimes even a bit of numbness. I also try not to overhydrate. I don't want to wash away all the minerals and vitamins that I take in. I find that if my pee is clear, I'm a bit overhydrated. I like to have a bit of color in my urine. (Does that qualify as too much information?)

After practice, I have an organic protein shake made from water mixed with rice or pea protein concentrate (which is sometimes called medical protein) and some evaporated cane juice. I don't drink whey or soy shakes. I find that, for me, this is the fastest way to replenish.

Before a match, when I really want to fire up, I usually eat a power gel with twenty-five milligrams of caffeine. But I'm careful—I never take more than that. It elevates my energy, but I don't want it to alter my concentration. Some people have the idea that five coffees or a big bottle of Coca-Cola will spike their energy. These folks will crash—and crash hard.

During a match, I eat dried fruits like dates. I have one or two teaspoons of honey. I always stick with sugars derived from fructose. Besides these examples, the vast majority of the sugar I consume comes from the training drinks I mentioned.

Later, when it's time for dinner, I eat protein in the form of meat or fish. That usually means steak, chicken, or salmon, as long as it's organic, grass-fed, free-range, wild, etc. I order meats roasted or grilled, and fish steamed or poached if possible. The closer the food is to nature, the more nutritious it is. I pair it with a steamed vegetable like zucchini or carrots. I may also have some chickpeas or lentils, or occasionally soup.

A lot of people also ask me about alcohol. I can't have beer or wheat-distilled vodka, so it's pointless to consider those. I never drink alcohol during a tournament. Period. Occasionally I have a glass of red wine. I don't consider it an alcoholic drink. I consider it a holy drink, something that can also be used as a curative. We've all heard about studies that show red wine is good for your heart. I don't drink much, however. For me, it creates an acidity in my digestive system, which can be uncomfortable.

Teas are wonderful any time of day. I like licorice tea, which gives me that wide-awake feeling without caffeine. It's also good for circulation. I also like a good ginger lemon tea.

A Week's Worth of Nutrition

You've just read a lot about my approach to food. My diet is always evolving, and I will never stop trying to improve it. This seven-day sample menu of gluten- and dairy-free foods is working well for me now, and I hope it will help you form your own menus. You'll find recipes for the italicized foods in chapter 8.

Monday

Breakfast

Water, first thing out of bed
2 tablespoons honey
Power Bowl Muesli with unsweetened almond milk or
    rice milk
Fruit

Midmorning snack (if needed)

Gluten-free bread or crackers with avocado and tuna

Lunch

Mixed-greens salad
Gluten-Free Pasta Primavera

Midafternoon snack

Apple with cashew butter
Cantaloupe, watermelon, or other melon

Dinner

Kale Caesar Salad with Quinoa
Minestrone soup
Simple Herbed Salmon

Tuesday

Breakfast

Water, first thing out of bed
2 tablespoons honey
Banana with cashew butter
Fruit

Midmorning snack (if needed)

Gluten-free toast with almond butter and honey

Lunch

Mixed-greens salad
Spicy Soba Noodle Salad

Midafternoon snack

Fruit and nut bar (such as a Kind bar)
Fruit

Dinner

Tuna Niçoise Salad
Tomato soup
Roasted Tomatoes

Wednesday

Breakfast

Water, first thing out of bed
2 tablespoons honey
Gluten-Free Oats with Cashew Butter and Bananas
Fruit

Midmorning snack (if needed)

Homemade Hummus with Apples/Crudités

Lunch

Mixed-greens salad
Gluten-Free Pasta with Power Pesto

Midafternoon snack

Avocado with gluten-free crackers
Fruit

Dinner

Fresh mixed-greens salad with avocado and homemade
    dressing
Carrot ginger soup
Whole Lemon-Roasted Chicken

Thursday

Breakfast

Water, first thing out of bed

2 tablespoons honey

Power Bowl Muesli with unsweetened almond milk or rice
milk

Fruit

Midmorning snack (if needed)

Apple and a handful of cashews or almonds

Lunch

Mixed-greens salad with quinoa, chicken, apples, avocado,
and homemade dressing

Midafternoon snack

Roasted Tamari Almonds

Fruit

Dinner

Fresh mixed-greens salad with avocado and homemade
dressing

Homemade Chicken Soup with Rice

Sea Bass with Mango and Papaya Salsa

Friday

Breakfast

Water, first thing out of bed
2 tablespoons honey
Banana with cashew butter
Fruit

Midmorning snack (if needed)

Gluten-free bread or crackers with tuna and hummus

Lunch

Mango Coconut Smoothie
Gluten-Free Pasta Primavera

Midafternoon snack

Fruit and nut bar (such as a Kind bar)
Fruit

Dinner

French onion soup
Fresh mixed-greens salad with quinoa, avocado, turkey
   breast, and homemade dressing

Saturday

Breakfast

Water, first thing out of bed
2 tablespoons honey
Gluten-Free Oats with Cashew Butter and Bananas

Midmorning snack (if needed)

Blueberry Almond Butter Smoothie

Lunch

Kale Caesar Salad with Quinoa

Midafternoon snack

Spiced beef jerky
Fruit

Dinner

Fresh mixed-greens salad with avocado and homemade
    dressing
Pea soup
Smoky Sirloin Steak
Loaded Baked Potatoes

Sunday

Breakfast
Water, first thing out of bed
2 tablespoons honey
Strawberry Banana Smoothie
Fruit

Midmorning snack (if needed)
Gluten-free toast with almond butter and honey

Lunch
Sun-Dried Tomato and Quinoa Salad

Midafternoon snack
Roasted Tamari Almonds
Fruit

Dinner
Fresh mixed-greens salad with avocado and homemade
    dressing
Tomato soup
Crispy Sweet Potato Fries
Bun-less Power Burger

CHAPTER 6

Training for the Mind

FOCUS TRAINING AND STRESS-BUSTING STRATEGIES FOR ACHIEVING EXCELLENCE

FOR ME, training isn't just about running myself ragged or repeating the same tennis skills over and over, year after year, until they're as familiar to my body as breathing. Well, okay, it's a lot about that. But not all. There are a lot of old and worn-out sayings in tennis, but this is one of my favorites: The game looks like it takes place between the lines on the court, but it really takes place between your ears.

This ties right in with everything I've been saying about food, because proper fuel doesn't power up only your body. During my struggles, before I discovered how to eat properly for my body, I didn't just stop performing physically at crucial moments. I was getting brain cramps as well as body cramps. Even in the most high-pressure situation imaginable, I was foggy and unfocused. You'd think that Rafael Nadal serving a ball in your direction at 145 miles per hour might be enough to keep your mind fully engaged, but I could tell that, mentally and emotionally, something wasn't right. The problem: what many doctors are now starting to call "grain brain."

Foods containing gluten have been linked to depression, lethargy, and even dementia and psychiatric disorders.[11] So you have to treat your mind the way you treat your body— you have to feed it properly.

But you also have to keep exercising it.

People often ask me, "How do you train for the mental game?" Well, as I said, I eat for my brain as well as my body. But there are also mental exercises you can do to help bring calm and clarity to your day. I won't give you all my secrets— I still want to have a career, after all—but I use a number of mental techniques to keep me sharp, focused, and dialed-in during both practice and matches. I don't necessarily think of them as "training methods," though.

They're how I live my life.

Flip Your Sign from "Closed" to "Open"

I talk a lot about open-mindedness and how my own attitudes have changed as I've traveled the world. But I want to

---

11. Numerous studies have linked both gluten and celiac disease to depression and other mental health issues. A 2006 study at the Mayo Clinic found a link between celiac disease and dementia and other forms of cognitive decline. SOURCE: *Archives of Neurology,* Josephs, KA et al., October 2006.

show you how a *lack* of open-mindedness in your everyday life affects how you feel and perform every single day.

For example, let's say you have a headache.

You say to a doctor, "I have a headache." He says, "Okay, we have something for that," and he gives you a pill that treats the symptoms but not the cause. This is the way Western medicine often operates. Forms of medicine from other cultures (Chinese, Ayurvedic) focus on treating the root cause instead. Sometimes the "cure" is as simple as a glass of water (dehydration can cause headaches, after all). But the Western doctor has his or her training and experience, and that's that. In my experience, most doctors who study one realm of Western medicine don't take time to familiarize themselves with alternative therapies—or even aspects of medicine outside their own specialties. Don't think for one second that I'm knocking Western medicine—trust me, if I blow out a knee and need surgery to reconstruct it, you can bet I'll be seeking out the best Western doctor I can find.

But this goes back to how I try to absorb and collect the experiences of people I meet from around the world and create a scenario that works for me. If everyone did that, we'd have a much happier, more peaceful world. *And* we'd all be healthier. Life is a work in progress, but progress happens only if you are open minded and open hearted. If you're not, then you can be easily manipulated.

I have touched on that idea already, but it bears more attention: People think that skepticism keeps them from being manipulated. The mindset today is all about being logical, rational, modern: "Give me proof that this works." And skepticism is often warranted: For example, the Internet gives us access to all sorts of "authoritative" information, but how can you trust its accuracy? Realize that every piece of "expert" advice has a backstory, and most people, even when they are genuinely trying to help you, are doing so in a way that also helps themselves. It's important to question both "proven" and new information—what do the sources have to gain?—without letting that skepticism close you to new ideas. As I said at the beginning of this book: Only you can be the ultimate authority on you. Sometimes you have to try new things and ask new questions to find your *own* proof: "Does this work *for me?*"

You know what that means? You have to objectively analyze yourself at that moment. That requires open-mindedness.

Not many people can, or are willing to, do that.

Let's go back to that headache example. A pill may be the fastest way to make the headache go away. But you're putting the pill into your body. Depending on which pill you take, you could be doing bad things to your liver or stomach. What if your headache comes back tonight? Or tomorrow? More pills? Meanwhile, if you're willing to be open minded and ask some questions, start with these:

How much water do I drink?
How much stress am I under?
And the biggest one of all: *What do I eat?*

Asking those three questions and improving those three issues could go a long way to reducing your headache without taking one pill. I mean, pill and supplement companies approach me all the time. There are pills and supplements for everything. But the answer doesn't lie in a pill.

It all comes down to awareness. I am dependent on my

body. You may think you're not as dependent on yours because you work in an office. But you are. You have to be at your best for your job. And at home? Don't people depend on you there? When it's not being cared for, your body will send you signals: fatigue, insomnia, cramps, flus, colds, allergies.

When that happens, will you ask yourself the questions that matter? Will you answer honestly and with an open mind?

I hope so. I've learned to do this, and now I know my own body well enough to be able to tell when something isn't right, and what I need to do to make it better. This openness is important, because it determines your energy. In my experience, open-minded people radiate positive energy. Closed-minded people radiate negativity. Remember that experiment with the water I told you about, where the water surrounded by negative energy turned foul?

Maybe you're starting to see what I'm talking about here.

Eastern medicine teaches you to align mind, body, and soul. If you have positive feelings in your mind—love, joy, happiness—they affect your body. I enjoy meeting crowds of people, especially if there are lots of kids around. Kids have nothing but positive energy. They're open to anything. They're enthusiastic, curious, waiting for another chance to laugh. I go out of my way to meet fans, sign autographs, and pose for pictures. Yes, it's a nice thing to do for them, but it also serves me well. I draw tremendous positive energy from crowds like that, and I need that positive energy to succeed. People who cheer for me, who stop me to say hi, have no idea how important they are to my success.

But a lot of people, especially closed-minded people, are led by fear. That and anger are the most negative energies we have. What are closed-minded people afraid of? It could be many things: Fear that they are wrong, fear that someone might have a better way, fear that something has to change. Fear limits your ability to live your life.

Another thing I get to see from my travels: Some people at the top feed off of negativity. The way I see it, pharmaceutical and food companies *want* people to feel fear. They *want* people to be sick. How many TV ads are for fast foods and medicines? And what's at the root of those messages? *We'll make you feel better with our products.* But even deeper down: *We'll make you fear that you don't have enough of the things we say you need.* It's crazy—even when you're completely healthy, they say you need supplements to stay that way.

Here's a pattern I'd rather embrace: good food, exercise, openness, positive energy, great results. I've been living that pattern for several years now. It works better than the alternative.

Don't be afraid to accept your own truth, to change, to analyze. Put questions in perspective. Try to be objective but not skeptical. And stay positive. That energy will fill your body and literally improve your health, fitness, and overall performance.

What Are You Thinking?

There is one important method I use to maintain that energy for myself, even when negative feelings creep in.

Emotionally, my "lows" are generally pretty high. Even

on days when I don't feel so great, once I start my routine, I get into it, and I hit every single ball with a purpose. So how do I keep my "lows" from bringing me down? The trick is all about how I think, or at least how I try to think most of the time. It's not absolute, or foolproof. But it works wonders.

Psychologists call it "mindfulness." It's a form of meditation where, instead of trying to silence your mind or find "inner peace," you allow and accept your thoughts as they come, objectively, without judging them, while being mindful of the moment in real time. The objectivity is key—it's how I get in touch with what's going on in my body in a given moment and how my thoughts have a direct effect on that. I can then analyze the thoughts without judging them. That process gives me clarity.

I do this every day for about fifteen minutes, and it is as important to me as my physical training. The practice is simple. Start by taking five minutes (set the alarm on your phone, if that helps). Just sit quietly, focus on your breathing, on the moment, and on the physical sensations you're feeling. Let your thoughts come. They do bounce around like crazy, let me tell you. But they're supposed to. Your job is to let them come and go. Try to remember that the physical sensations you're experiencing are real, but the thoughts in your head aren't—they're just made up. Your goal is to learn to separate the two.

Silence is a big part of this exercise. And as I mentioned, I now like to eat slowly, quietly, for much the same reason. This is all part of how I try to deliver both good food and positive energy to my body as I fuel up. There is so much urgent noise in our lives that's designed to bring on stress. Mindfulness is a way to back out of that and just . . . be.

If you do this regularly, even for short chunks of time, you learn amazing things about yourself because you're being mindful of the moment and, finally, *noticing*. For me, I realized just how much negative energy I have coursing through my brain. Once I focused on taking a step back and looking at my thoughts objectively, I saw it plainly: a massive amount of negative emotion. Self-doubt. Anger. Worries about my life, my family. Fears about not being good enough. That my training is wrong. That my approach to a coming match is wrong. That I'm wasting time, wasting potential. And then there are the little battles: the imaginary arguments you have with people you won't even see that day over subjects that will never come up.

You might think, *Why would I want to dredge up all that ugliness? It sounds horrible.* But it's not. It's liberating. Understand, I'm not holding on to these thoughts. I'm letting them come and then go. And because I'm mindful of the moment, I see how dwelling on this energy takes the life out of me.

After practicing meditation for a while, something clicked: This is simply how my mind works. It's probably how everyone's mind works. I wasted a lot of energy and time on my own "inner turmoil," or however you want to describe it. I was so focused on this inner battle that I lost sight of what was happening around me, what was going on in the moment.

I've done so much mindful meditation that now my brain functions better automatically, even when I'm not meditating. I used to freeze up whenever I made a mistake; I was sure that I wasn't in the same league as the Federers and the Andy Murrays. Now, when I blow a serve or shank a backhand, I still get those flashes of self-doubt, but I know how to handle them: I acknowledge the negative thoughts and let them slide by, focusing on the moment. That mindfulness helps me process pain and emotions. It lets me focus on what's really important. It helps me turn down the volume in my brain. Imagine how handy that is for me in the middle of a Grand Slam championship match. That's why mindfulness has helped shape one of my driving philosophies in sport: If you can focus on this match, on this day, as the most important thing right now, then the result will be the best possible.

A lot of people ask, "How do you meditate? It seems so strange." It's really simple. Start small, with brief chunks of time. You don't have to cross your legs and burn incense and chant "om." You can just sit quietly, focusing on your breathing, or go for a walk outside, focusing on each step as you go. The goal isn't to see how long you can do it. It's not an endurance event. The goal of meditation is to find calm, focus, and positive energy.

The greatest challenge when first trying it out is allowing ourselves "me" time. It seems like we give less and less time to ourselves, but are happy to dedicate more time to all the other distractions that raise our stress, not lower it. I used to think I needed to be "busy" every moment of the day, but again, with an open mind, I learned to set aside the time I need. My meals are sacred time. I cherish silence when I can find it (and sometimes I force the issue and disappear for a quick break).

To make this work for you, discover the time within your

time, like cracks in your day. Have a healthy meal, or step out for fresh air. Don't think you're being "selfish" or "lazy" or some other stupid label when you take some quiet time. A lot of people assume that when you're not busy, you're wasting time, being useless or lazy. That's what I felt before I began cherishing and respecting this time.

It helps to be vigilant for opportunities. Let's say you have kids, and you're watching them all day. Suddenly, all three kids are occupied, and you have ten minutes for yourself. Instead of thinking, "I have to do $x, y, z \ldots$," try to use this time to be in the moment with your thoughts. Acknowledge them. Then let them go.

The more you practice, the better you'll get. Soon this time will feel vital to your day. And after that, you'll feel the changes in how you think all day long. The negative energy will slip by. The positive energy will dominate.

You'll feel amazing.

The Most Important Part of My Day

. . . is night.

Specifically, the moment when my head hits the pillow. I'm serious. I treat sleep with as much respect as I treat food, or my training schedule, or my rivals. It's that important.

Most people disrespect sleep. I see it a lot. I read one statistic that said at least one out of four people don't get enough sleep. And if you're one of those people, I bet you feel it every day.

Here's why I never skimp on sleep: Exercise and sleep are like a married couple that never fights. They complement each other. How? A good night's sleep helps you have a stronger workout. A stronger workout improves your sleep quality. You train to improve your body, and sleep allows your body to recover so it's stronger tomorrow. Let exercise help you sleep better; let sleep help you exercise better.

People either forget this or ignore it. (And if you're hearing it for the first time right now, I hope you listen!) In fact, among the three major habits that can ensure good health—eating right and exercising being the first two—sleep probably gets ignored most frequently. If you eat something lousy or skip a workout, you (maybe) feel bad about it, or at the very least acknowledge your shortcoming. But if you lose a few hours of sleep? Even every night? You chalk it up to being busy. Being busy is important. No one ever feels bad about being busy. But not being busy? That's scary.

But take a look at sleep and how it helps an active body, and hopefully you'll change your tune.

There are four stages of sleep. The first two are transition phases from wakefulness, and typically take just a few minutes each. But once you reach the third stage, the really deep sleep, you release growth hormone, which helps rebuild muscle and repair stress damage. Stage four is REM sleep, when you dream, and it helps improve learning and cognition. You cycle through these stages four to six times per night. Your body needs every one of them, uninterrupted.

You need to have only one lousy night's sleep to know you're doing something unhealthy to your body. Think about it. When you're sleep deprived, are you full of positive energy? Of course not. Do you crave salad? No, you want lousy comfort food, and tons of it. When you're sleep deprived and try to work out, how does it go? You skimp on the workout, or go more slowly than normal, or just skip it completely.

Now run through those same scenarios when you've had a full night's rest. You feel terrific, are motivated to eat like a champion, and are mentally and physically prepared to have a great workout. The positive cycle begins because the great workout helps make the next night's sleep even better.

Now, all that said, a lot of things conspire to mess up my sleep patterns. I travel. I change time zones. And sometimes I have to sleep in smaller doses than I'd like. I take that sleep whenever and wherever I can get it. But I also use some tricks to help make sure the sleep I get is the best quality it can be.

1. **I keep a routine whenever humanly possible.** I try to go to bed at the same time every night—between 11 and midnight—and get up at the same time every morning—about 7 A.M.—even on weekends. This keeps my body clock accurate. It exposes me to a regular pattern of light and dark, and helps my body adjust to a new time zone. When I keep this schedule, everything feels in sync and my training improves.

2. **I don't bother with caffeine.** I've admitted to an energy gel before a match, but that's the extent of it. Alcohol and caffeine both work against your body's ability to regulate its inner clock.

3. **I wind down with useful activities.** The time right before you go to sleep is great for mindful meditation. Your home is at its most quiet. Doing a few yoga stretches right before bed feels good, too. Sometimes I read. My girlfriend, Jelena, and I both keep diaries,

and we use the quiet time in the evening to write down our thoughts and reflect on the day.

4. **I shut out the world.** Some of my friends and family have tried soothing sound machines for sleep and had good results. These can help you tune out neighborhood noise, the TV downstairs, or any other disturbances so you can fall asleep and stay asleep. Ear plugs and eye shades help, too, especially on long plane rides.

5. **If I wake up before I should, I stay put.** I used to stress about this, lying there staring at the ceiling getting angry that I was missing my sleep. Sometimes I'd get up and do chores. Now, I use this time for mindful meditation. That either helps me get back to sleep or keeps me from stressing about the sleeplessness.

6. **I use melatonin supplements.** Melatonin is a naturally occurring hormone that helps your body recover from jet lag and regain its circadian rhythm after long flights. Most of the professional players I know swear by it.

7. **When I wake up in the morning, I seek the sun.** I pull up the shades and let the light in. Sometimes I step outside to feel the sun on my face. It makes me feel more awake. The light lets my body and brain know that it's time to go to work.

My Secret Weapon—Friendships

I've been very successful, and as strange as this may sound, success can draw out nasty, negative energy, both in myself and in others. One subject that always comes up in a discussion about success is money. At every tournament, tennis commentators and sportswriters love to talk about the total purse and prize breakdown: "If he wins today, he collects X dollars, or Y euros, or Z what-have-you."

I try to be positive about the negative aspects of money, but I'm also honest about its importance in life. I am very aware of what money represents, and that life can be much easier if you have it in bigger amounts. It saves me time, for one—I don't have to worry about paying bills or putting food on the table. I enjoy some creature comforts. My family also can have the house, the cars, the basic things we didn't have before. But it's not everything. I know that and I focus on that. My friends and family make sure that the spoils of my success don't spoil me.

Which leads me to another key force that keeps driving me in a positive direction, a factor that eliminates much of the stress money and success bring: the people around me.

I'm very careful about the people I have around me. I spend almost every waking moment with my physiotherapist, my manager, and my coaches. My girlfriend is with me most of the time, and my parents often are as well. These people are very modest, humble, normal people who lead normal lives. They've also been through a lot of good and bad experiences. They are present to give me that extra hand, that extra support. Whenever I am in a tough moment, I can rely on them for their experience, their wisdom, and their consolation.

This is extremely important. People think of tennis as an individual sport, one person facing a foe across the net.

That's the literal interpretation, but no. It's a team effort. Everything I have achieved has been a team effort. Everybody does their job, and we all work in harmony and understand what everyone else is doing, and why. I have to work this way. It helps to build team spirit, a driving force behind success.

I think of the people around me as family (and some literally are), and we think of our relationships as friendships first, professional partnerships afterward. I cannot work differently. I need to connect with the people around me, to be able to share my thoughts, good and bad, and all the big feelings in life: happiness and joy, worry and stress.

These people have another big job: They make sure I remain the same guy, with the same philosophies and character, that I've always been. They don't let me forget who I am and where I grew up. That's their mission, and they take it seriously.

Recently my trainer, Miljan, gave me a big compliment. He said, "Two years ago, you won all those tournaments— the Grand Slams, all of it—and you've kept winning since then, but your biggest achievement is that you didn't change. You stayed the same guy."

He'd better say those things to me. I'm godfather to his daughter.

I joke, but you can see we have much more than a trainer/ player relationship. He's one of my best friends. That's invaluable to me.

Perhaps you noticed Winston Churchill's quote at the beginning of this book: "We make a living by what we get, but we make a life by what we give." So as much as you give to the people around you, that's how much your soul grows, and how much you grow as a human being.

Love, joy, happiness, and health: Those are the things I always look out for and try to never take for granted. I always want to be aware of myself, of life, and of the people and world around me.

That's the best kind of mindfulness, isn't it?

All of those things contribute to my success, but there is one other thing that drives me: the hope that others coming after me can see what I've done, and how I've done it, and use my work to fuel their own achievements. That alone is huge motivation for me to remain positive and stay my course. I always try to stay humble, but I also know that I became what I am today from nothing, and that was no easy task. I came from a place that was torn by war, during a time of food shortages, restrictions, sanctions, and embargoes. There was no tennis tradition whatsoever, and no money for my family to send me to tournaments, yet I still grew up to become number one in the world.

Because of that, nobody can ever tell me, "It's impossible." It seemed impossible at the time, believe me. Very few people believed that I could make it. Today, I'm fortunate to be around those people who did believe in me and allowed me to become what I am. That's why I say, "Who you're with is who you are." Think about that—and everything in this chapter—as you try to achieve your own success. Those beliefs are my foundations for living.

Maintaining focus can be excruciatingly hard. Everybody deals with stress, nervousness, and frustration: I'm not feeling good today, so screw this or screw that. It's normal because you are human. But remember: The amount of control you have over yourself to overcome those feelings determines your quality of life. My quality of life is formed by the people that I have around me, and my love for them; they remind me every day to focus on what's important, and to set aside my frustrations and fears. If my career disappears tomorrow, and my friends and family are all I have left, well, that's more than enough.

CHAPTER 7

Training for the Body

A SIMPLE FITNESS PLAN ANYONE CAN LIVE BY

AM AWAKE for about sixteen hours a day, and probably fourteen of those hours are spent (a) playing tennis, (b) training to play tennis, or (c) eating so I can be better at tennis. It is all that I do, every day, for eleven months out of the year—that's how long the professional tennis season is. (During my few weeks off in the beginning of May, I still spend most of my time doing a, b, and c, but I also take time to do a lot of hiking, kayaking, and bike riding.)

This is what it takes to be number one against the fittest and most competitive athletes in the world: constant, unyielding mental and physical preparation, fourteen hours a day, seven days a week.

So, ready to get started?

No?

That makes sense. My physical needs probably don't translate very closely to yours. (And if they do, you likely have your own trainers and coaches and are playing me next weekend in Paris.)

Still, I want to show you some of the exercises I do that could make a big difference in your life. These are not whole workouts. They are little things you can add to your current workout plan, and they'll help anyone at any fitness level. Understand, the dietary changes suggested in this book will have you feeling better and better. You should take advantage of them to raise your physical game, whatever that may be. Then, whether you like distance running or power lifting or maybe even tennis (I, of course, recommend it), these exercise tips will help you.

They aren't just about becoming fitter, though they help with that. They also promote better performance because, for example, they help your body warm up more effectively before a workout. They promote flexibility. They control stress. And they are also terrific for one very important facet of training that's overlooked: recovery.

The bottom line: These exercises give me an edge. I wouldn't be able to play at my current level without them.

Achieve "Real" Flexibility

For me, every practice, every workout, every match starts the same way: ten to fifteen minutes of movement. That's running or biking in the fitness center, followed by dynamic stretching on the sidelines. None of this is too intense—it's just to warm up my muscles. If I'm on the bike, it's set on level 1 or 2. Because I must be extremely aware of the potential for injury, I don't play even a fun exhibition charity match without a proper warm-up. Safety first.

Next I do dynamic stretching, which really wakes up my body. If you're not familiar with this term, understand that there are two kinds of stretching: static and dynamic. Static stretching is what we did as kids in gym class, which is to hold a stretch for thirty seconds. That doesn't help me much. Once I learned dynamic stretches (which I explain in detail on the coming pages), I could feel that my body was truly ready for a good workout. I could also feel a new kind of effortless flexibility.

To me, "real" or "true" flexibility isn't whether I can reach down and touch my toes (though I can). It's not about being a contortionist. It's about whether my body can execute the movements I need to win. Dynamic stretching helps get me there because "dynamic," or movement-based, stretching is all about real-world actions. That's why I love it: It makes everything I do easier. Dynamic stretching also stimulates your central nervous system and increases blood flow as well as strength and power production. So, really, it's the ideal warm-up for any activity.

My recommendation: Do five minutes of light jogging or stationary cycling to ease your body into activity and raise your heart rate. Then go right into these dynamic stretching exercises. Do ten reps of each without resting (as your body becomes conditioned to these moves, you can increase the reps to fifteen or even twenty). It shouldn't take you more than five minutes to run through them, and once you do, you should be sweating. That's a good thing—you're putting the warm in warm-up.

Jumping jacks. You probably know how to do them, but if not: Stand with your feet together and your hands at your sides. In one simultaneous movement, raise your arms above your head and jump up enough to spread your feet wide, then quickly reverse the movement and repeat.

Walking high knees. Stand with your feet shoulder-width apart. Keeping your shoulders back and your back straight, raise your left knee as high as you can and step forward. Repeat with your right leg. Continue to alternate back and forth.

Walking high kicks. Stand with your feet shoulder-width apart. Keeping your knee straight, kick your right leg up and reach out with your left arm to meet it—as you simultaneously take a step forward. As soon as your right foot touches the floor, repeat the movement with your left leg and right arm. Alternate back and forth.

Squat thrusts (a.k.a. burpees). Stand with your feet shoulder-width apart and your arms at your sides. Lower your body as deep as you can into a squat. As you squat down, place your hands on the floor in front of you, shifting your weight onto them. Kick your legs backward, so that you're now in a push-up position. Quickly bring your legs back to the squat position. Stand up and repeat.

Lunge with side bend. From a standing position, step forward with your right leg and lower your body until your right knee is bent at least ninety degrees (don't let your left knee touch the ground). As you lunge, reach over your head with your left arm as you bend your torso sideways to your right. Reach for the floor with your right hand if you need extra balance. Return to the starting position.

Complete your reps, then switch legs for the same number of reps.

Reverse lunge with backward reach. From a standing position, step back with your right leg, lowering your body until your left knee is bent at least ninety degrees (don't let your right knee touch the ground). As you lunge, keep your torso facing forward, but reach your arms back over your shoulders and to the left. Reverse the movement to come back to the starting position.

Complete your reps, then step back with your left leg and reach over your right shoulder for the same number of reps.

Low side-to-side lunge. Stand with your feet about twice shoulder-width apart, facing straight ahead. Clasp your hands in front of your chest.

Shift your weight to your right leg and lower your body by dropping your hips and bending your right knee. Your lower left leg should be nearly parallel to the floor. Your right foot should remain flat on the floor.

Without raising yourself back up to a standing position, reverse the movement to the left. Alternate back and forth.

Inverted hamstring. Stand on your left leg, your knee bent slightly. Raise your right foot slightly off the floor. Your arms should be at your sides. Without changing the angle in your left knee, bend at your hips and lower your torso until it's parallel to the floor and your right leg is extended out behind you.

As you bend over, raise your arms straight out from your

sides until they're at shoulder level, your palms facing down. Your right leg should stay in line with your body as you lower your torso.

Return to the start. Complete the reps on your left leg, then do the same number on your right.

Inchworm. Stand with your legs straight, and while keeping them straight, bend over and brace your hands on the floor (you may have to bend your legs to do this, but do the best you can). Walk your hands forward as far as you can without allowing your hips to sag. When your body is stretched out, pause, then take small steps with your feet toward your hands as your butt rises back into the air and your body pikes. The entire motion mimics an inchworm. That's one repetition. Do five forward, and then five more in reverse. To reverse the movement, bend over and brace your hands on the floor, then walk your feet backward as far as you can. Once you're stretched out, pause and slowly walk your hands back toward your feet as your butt rises and your body pikes.

Get on a Roll

For a tennis player, recovery is the ultimate goal—you may come off a grueling four-hour match at 11 P.M. and need to play another one the next afternoon. So I get some level of massage almost every day to help my muscles recover and my body to process the toxins that build up during a long match or training session. I think of massage as a necessity, not a luxury. For most people, it's the opposite, and I understand that because of the expense. But if you can invest in a professional massage even once a month, you'll see long-term rewards.

It's not just that your muscles "get tight." There's more going on in there than muscles tearing, repairing, and re-tearing. For example, massage is an important way to keep your fascia as supple as possible. Fascia is a tough substance that runs around and through your muscles and connective tissue. It acts as both support and shock absorber. (Think of cutting through a raw chicken breast: That thin, white plastic wrap–like layer around it is the fascia.) If it tightens up, your muscles can't function properly, and you could wind up with pain or injury. A regular massage can help keep your muscles—and the fascia in and around them—loose and healthy.

But here's an interesting idea: What if you could give yourself a massage every single day for a one-time price of around $20?

That leads me to another important part of my overall training: foam rolling. Foam rollers are available in any sporting goods shop, and they're nothing more than a hard Styrofoam roll, usually about three feet long. You "foam roll" by rolling different parts of your body over the tube, in effect giving yourself a massage. You'll loosen tough connective tissue (like the fascia) and decrease the stiffness of your muscles. The result? Better flexibility and mobility, and muscles that can function properly. And you can foam-roll anytime, even while talking on the phone. (Traveling and don't have a roller? Use a tennis ball!)

If you've never foam-rolled before, I should warn you: It can be excruciating. But every trainer I know says that if an area really hurts, that's where you need to work. It means a certain muscle is tight and needs attention. And the good part is that the more you do it, the less intense it feels because you're making the muscle more supple.

So how do you do it? It's simple: For each muscle that you work, slowly move it back and forth over the roller for thirty seconds. If you hit a really tender spot, pause on it for five to ten seconds. That's it.

Hamstrings roll. Place a foam roller under your right knee, with your leg straight. Cross your left leg over your right ankle. Put your hands flat on the floor for support. Keep your back naturally arched.

Roll your body forward until the roller reaches your glutes. Then roll back and forth. Repeat with the roller under your left thigh. If rolling one leg is too difficult, perform the movement with both legs on the roller.

Glutes roll. Sit on a foam roller with it positioned on the back of your right thigh, just below your glutes. Cross your right ankle over the front of your left thigh. Put your hands flat on the floor for support.

Roll your body forward until the roller reaches your lower back. Then roll back and forth. Repeat with the roller under your left glute.

Iliotibial-band roll. Your iliotibial band—called the IT band—is a tough strip of connective tissue that runs down the side of your thigh, starting on your hip bone and connecting just below your knee. A tight IT band can cause bursitis in your hip or pain in your knee.

Lie on your left side and place your left hip on a foam roller, with the roller perpendicular to your leg. Put your hands on the floor in front of you for support. Cross your right leg over your left and place your right foot flat on the floor.

Roll your body upward, adjusting your hands as needed, until the roller reaches your knee. Then roll up and down. Lie on your right side and repeat with the roller under your right hip. (If this becomes too easy over time, place your right leg on top of your left instead of bracing it on the floor.)

Calf roll. Place a foam roller under your right ankle, with your right leg straight, the roller perpendicular to your leg. Cross your left leg over your right ankle. Put your hands flat on the floor for support and keep your back naturally arched.

Roll your body forward until the roller reaches the back of your right knee. Then roll up and down. Repeat with the roller under your left calf. (If this is too hard, perform the movement with both legs on the roller.)

Quadriceps and hip flexors roll. Lie facedown on the floor with a foam roller positioned above your right knee, perpendicular to your leg. Cross your left leg over your right ankle and place your elbows on the floor for support.

Roll your body backward until the roller reaches the top of your right thigh. Then roll up and down. Repeat with the roller under your left thigh. (If that's too hard, perform the movement with both thighs on the roller.)

Groin roll. Not as much fun as it sounds. Lie facedown on the floor, supported by your elbows. Place a foam roller beside you, parallel to your body. Raise your right thigh until it's nearly perpendicular to your body, with the inner portion of your thigh, just above the level of your knee, resting on top of the roller.

Roll your body toward the right until the roller reaches your pelvis. Then roll back and forth. Repeat with the roller under your left thigh.

Lower-back roll. Lie faceup with a foam roller under your mid-back. Cross your arms over your chest. Your knees should be bent, with your feet flat on the floor. Raise your hips off the floor slightly. Roll back and forth over your lower back.

Upper-back roll. Lie faceup with a foam roller under your mid-back, at the bottom of your shoulder blades. Clasp your hands behind your head and pull your elbows toward each other. Raise your hips off the floor slightly.

Slowly move so your upper back bends over the foam roller. Return to the starting position and roll forward a couple of inches—so that the roller sits higher under your upper back—and repeat. Do it again. That's one rep.

Shoulder-blades roll. Lie faceup with a foam roller under your upper back, at the tops of your shoulder blades. Cross your arms over your chest. Your knees should be bent with your feet flat on the floor.

Raise your hips off the floor slightly. Roll back and forth over your shoulder blades and your mid- and upper back.

Push Your Body *and* Your Mind

I use yoga for a variety of reasons. It helps me stay loose, for one. Sometimes my back and hips stiffen up, and yoga is an amazing remedy for that. The breathing sequences also help me clear my mind. A few years ago, I did yoga on a daily basis, but now I use it to supplement the training I'm already doing, especially between tournaments. If my body tells me that I'm a little tight, or if I feel more stress than I'd like, I do a yoga session.

Yoga is an ancient practice, so millions of people over thousands of years can't be wrong. I've put in a brief routine here with some very basic moves, but you can delve much deeper into the practice. I recommend that everyone find a good yoga class and attend regularly. (I know that some guys out there might be skeptical, but it really is seriously good stuff for athleticism and flexibility. Most elite athletes I know use it on some level.)

I use moves based on four animals: rabbit, cat, dog, and cobra. These four moves stretch most of my body and create a very relaxing routine. The perfect time to try this routine is right after a workout, or in the evening before bed, for the de-stressing benefits as well as the flexibility.

Hold each *asana,* or pose, for thirty seconds to one minute, breathing deeply and slowly through your nose. *Breathing is the key.* Beginners should make adjustments for moves that are too challenging for now (you'll get better).

Rabbit: You might know this as "child's pose." Start on your hands and knees with your back straight, your hips over your knees and your shoulders over your wrists. Sit back, moving your butt all the way to your heels. Straighten your arms and press your forehead to the floor. (Use your hands to push your body back until your butt meets your heels.)

Cat: From the Rabbit position, return to the starting position, on your hands and knees. Arch your spine toward the ceiling like a cat, exhaling as your press your palms into the floor and drop your tailbone down.

Dog: This pose is better known as the "downward facing dog." Return to the starting position on your hands and knees. Now walk your hands a few inches in front of your shoulders. Curl your toes under, lift your hips, and straighten your legs. Keeping your arms straight, press down into the floor with all ten fingers and your palms. Extend your heels away from your toes and try to push them to the floor.

Cobra: From the Dog position, shift your weight forward so your chest is over your hands, and simultaneously lower your hips so you wind up in a push-up position. Slowly bend your elbows and lower your body to the floor. Your palms should be next to your ribs. Rest for a moment. Press all ten toes into the floor, and press your palms into the floor to lift your head and chest, bringing your ribs and belly off the floor so there's a slight arch in your back. Draw back the tops of your shoulders to broaden your upper chest. You should be looking straight ahead, or slightly upward.

CHAPTER 8

The Champion's Plate

RECIPES THAT FUEL MY SUCCESS

THERE IS NO SHORTAGE of gluten-free, dairy-free foods available today, even in mainstream restaurants and grocery stores. But as I've said, no matter where I travel, I look for hotel rooms that have their own kitchens. I always feel better when I know exactly what I'm eating, and my family and I get to spend a lot of time cooking and eating together.

These recipes all fit perfectly with my eating recommendations. They were developed by author and chef Candice Kumai, who kindly created them based on my eating habits—which happen to be the same as hers!

Whether you choose to make these recipes, cook your own family favorites, or just order in, remember that how you eat is as important as what you eat. And take what you put into your body seriously, because it will soon *be* your body.

Recipes

Breakfast
Power Bowl Muesli

Gluten-Free Oats with Cashew Butter and Bananas

Smoothies
Blueberry Almond Butter Smoothie

Strawberry Banana Smoothie

Mango Coconut Smoothie

Chocolate Almond Butter Smoothie

Vanilla Almond Smoothie

Lunch
Gluten-Free Pasta with Power Pesto

Gluten-Free Pasta Primavera

Spicy Soba Noodle Salad

Sun-Dried Tomato and Quinoa Salad

Snacks
Roasted Tamari Almonds

Homemade Hummus with Apples/Crudités

Dinner
Sea Bass with Mango and Papaya Salsa

Roasted Tomatoes

Kale Caesar Salad with Quinoa

Whole Lemon-Roasted Chicken

Simple Herbed Salmon

Smoky Sirloin Steak

Loaded Baked Potatoes

Bun-less Power Burger

Crispy Sweet Potato Fries

Tuna Niçoise Salad

Homemade Chicken Soup with Rice

Breakfast

Power Bowl Muesli

SERVES 2

Ingredients:

1 cup organic gluten-free rolled oats
½ cup dried cranberries
½ cup golden raisins
½ cup pepitas (pumpkin seeds) or sunflower seeds
½ cup sliced almonds
Rice or almond milk (optional)
Bananas, berries, or sliced apples (optional)
Natural sweetener (optional)

Directions:

1. Combine the oats, cranberries, raisins, seeds, and almonds in a medium bowl or, if traveling, a resealable plastic bag.
2. Serve with rice or almond milk; bananas, berries, or sliced apples; and your favorite natural sweetener, if desired.

Gluten-Free Oats with Cashew Butter and Bananas

SERVES 4

Ingredients:

2 cups organic gluten-free rolled oats
2 firm but ripe bananas, thinly sliced on the bias
3 tablespoons natural cashew butter or almond butter
1 tablespoon brown sugar
¼ cup chopped dark chocolate (optional)
Rice milk or unsweetened almond milk (optional)

Directions:

1. Bring 4 cups water to a boil in a medium saucepan, stir in the oats, and cook for 3 to 5 minutes, to the desired consistency. Ladle the oatmeal into 4 bowls.
2. Distribute the bananas on top of the oatmeal. Top each bowl with one quarter of the cashew butter, brown sugar, and dark chocolate, if using. Add rice milk or almond milk if desired.

Smoothies

Blueberry Almond Butter Smoothie

SERVES 4

Ingredients:

2 cups frozen blueberries
1 frozen banana
2 tablespoons almond butter
1 cup fresh spinach
2 cups unsweetened almond milk

Directions:

In a blender, puree the blueberries, banana, almond butter, spinach, and almond milk until fully combined. (If necessary, stop the blender to scrape the sides with a spatula, then reblend until smooth.) Pour into 4 glasses and serve immediately.

Strawberry Banana Smoothie

SERVES 4

Ingredients:

2 cups frozen strawberries
1 frozen banana
1 tablespoon almond butter
1 cup fresh spinach
2 cups unsweetened almond milk

Directions:

In a large blender, puree the strawberries, banana, almond butter, spinach, and unsweetened almond milk until fully combined.* Pour into 4 glasses and serve immediately.

*If needed, stop the blender safely, scrape the sides of the blender with a spatula, and reblend to combine.

Mango Coconut Smoothie

SERVES 4

Ingredients:

2 cups frozen mango
1 frozen banana
1 tablespoon almond butter
1 tablespoon shredded coconut
1 cup kale leaves, stems removed
2 cups rice milk

Directions:

In a large blender, puree the mango, banana, almond butter, shredded coconut, kale leaves, and rice milk. Blend until fully combined.* Pour into 4 glasses and serve immediately.

*If needed, stop the blender safely, scrape the sides of the blender with a spatula, and reblend to combine.

Chocolate Almond Butter Smoothie

SERVES 4

Ingredients:

3 frozen bananas
2 tablespoons organic chocolate syrup
2 tablespoons almond butter
1 cup kale leaves, stems removed
½ cup ice
1½ cups unsweetened almond milk

Directions:

In a large blender, puree the bananas, chocolate syrup, almond butter, kale leaves, ice, and almond milk. Blend until fully combined.* Pour into 4 glasses and serve immediately.

*If needed, stop the blender safely, scrape the sides of the blender with a spatula, and reblend to combine.

Vanilla Almond Smoothie

SERVES 4

Ingredients:

3 frozen bananas
2 tablespoons almond butter
1 teaspoon organic vanilla extract
1 tablespoon honey
1 cup fresh spinach
½ cup ice (or as needed)
1½ cups unsweetened almond milk

Directions:

In a large blender, puree the bananas, almond butter, vanilla extract, honey, spinach, ice, and almond milk. Blend until fully combined.* Pour into 4 glasses and serve immediately.

*If needed, stop the blender safely, scrape the sides of the blender with a spatula, and reblend to combine.

Lunch

Gluten-Free Pasta with Power Pesto

SERVES 4

Ingredients:

3 cups loosely packed fresh basil leaves, plus more for
   garnish, if desired
¾ cup roughly chopped walnuts
3 garlic cloves, roughly chopped
½ teaspoon sea salt
½ cup extra-virgin olive oil
2 tablespoons fresh lemon juice
5 cups rice pasta
Chopped sun-dried tomatoes (optional)

Directions:

1. To make the pesto, place the basil, walnuts, garlic, and sea
   salt in a food processor and pulse to combine until the
   ingredients are somewhat mealy. Gradually add the olive
   oil in a steady stream, processing until the mixture is finely
   chopped yet still has texture, about 1 minute. Pulse in the
   lemon juice and adjust the seasoning to taste. Transfer to a
   large bowl.
2. In a medium saucepan, cook the rice pasta according to
   package instructions. Strain, reserving some of the pasta
   water. Toss with the pesto until well coated, thinning as
   needed with the reserved pasta water. Top with additional
   basil and sun-dried tomatoes, if desired.

Gluten-Free Pasta Primavera

SERVES 4

Ingredients:

2 tablespoons extra-virgin olive oil

2 garlic cloves, finely minced

1 yellow summer squash, halved lengthwise and thinly sliced into half-moons

1 zucchini, halved lengthwise and thinly sliced into half-moons

½ bunch (½ pound) asparagus, trimmed and sliced on the bias

4 cups rice pasta

¼ cup thinly sliced sun-dried tomatoes, plus more for garnish, if desired

¼ teaspoon sea salt

2 tablespoons grated vegan cheese, to top (optional)

Chopped fresh herbs, such as parsley or basil (optional)

Directions:

1. In a large sauté pan over medium heat, combine the olive oil and garlic and cook until fragrant, about 5 minutes.
2. Add the sliced squash, zucchini, and asparagus and sauté until tender, stirring occasionally, about 8 minutes.
3. Meanwhile, cook the pasta in a large pot according to package instructions. Strain the cooked pasta and return to the pot.
4. When the vegetables are tender, add them to the pasta and toss well to combine. Stir in the sun-dried tomatoes and sea salt. If desired, top with vegan cheese to taste and serve with fresh herbs and additional sun-dried tomatoes.

Spicy Soba Noodle Salad

SERVES 4

Ingredients:

1 8-ounce package gluten-free soba noodles
1 red bell pepper, halved, seeded, and thinly sliced
1 cup arugula
2 tablespoons crushed cashews
2 tablespoons chopped fresh basil leaves
Lime wedges (optional)

For the spicy vinaigrette:
2 tablespoons creamy organic peanut butter
1 teaspoon reduced-sodium soy sauce
2 tablespoons roasted sesame oil
2 tablespoons rice vinegar
2 teaspoons hot sauce, like sriracha or Tabasco
1 teaspoon agave nectar or honey

Directions:

1. Cook the soba noodles as directed on the package. Drain and rinse under cool water. Set aside.
2. While the soba is cooking, combine all the vinaigrette ingredients in a large bowl. Whisk well to combine.
3. In the same large mixing bowl, gently toss the cooled soba noodles in the vinaigrette, coating them well. Add the red pepper and arugula.
4. Top the noodles with the cashews and basil. Add a squeeze of lime if desired.

Sun-Dried Tomato and Quinoa Salad

SERVES 4

Ingredients:

For the dressing:
2 tablespoons extra-virgin olive oil
3 tablespoons balsamic vinegar
1 teaspoon honey
½ teaspoon sea salt
1 teaspoon Dijon mustard

For the salad:
4 cups cooked, cooled quinoa
½ cup oil-packed sun-dried tomatoes,* thinly sliced
½ cup basil leaves, torn
¼ cup pine nuts
1 cup arugula

Directions:

1. In a large mixing bowl, whisk together the olive oil, vinegar, honey, sea salt, and Dijon mustard until combined.
2. Add the quinoa, sun-dried tomatoes, basil, pine nuts, and arugula. Toss to coat evenly with the dressing.

   *To save on calories, opt for reconstituting dry sun-dried tomatoes in water.

Snacks

Roasted Tamari Almonds

SERVES 6

Ingredients:

4 cups raw almonds
2 tablespoons coconut oil, melted
2 tablespoons tamari (gluten-free soy sauce)
2 tablespoons dried oregano
2 teaspoons garlic powder

To finish:
½ teaspoon chili powder
1 teaspoon garlic powder
½ teaspoon fine sea salt

Directions:

1. Preheat the oven to 350°F. Line two baking sheets with foil, evenly spread the almonds on the pans, and roast for about 8 minutes. Remove from the oven and cool slightly. Lower the oven temperature to 300°F.
2. In a large mixing bowl, combine the coconut oil, tamari, oregano, and garlic powder. Add the almonds and mix until well coated.
3. Place the coated almonds back on the baking sheets, return to the oven, and roast for about 8 more minutes, stirring and rotating the pans halfway through.

4. In a small bowl, combine the chili powder, garlic powder, and sea salt. Remove the almonds from the oven and cool slightly. To finish, sprinkle with the dry mixture and toss to coat. Store in an airtight container for up to 2 weeks.

Homemade Hummus with Apples/Crudités

SERVES 12

Ingredients:

For the hummus:

2 15-ounce cans garbanzo beans, rinsed and drained
2 tablespoons extra-virgin olive oil
2 tablespoons tahini paste (optional)
Juice of ½ lemon
4 roasted garlic cloves
1 teaspoon ground cumin
2 tablespoons tamari (gluten-free soy sauce)

For dipping:

4 large apples (preferably a sweet-crisp one like Fuji), halved,
   cored, and sliced into wedges

Directions:

Place all the ingredients for the hummus in a food processor and blend until smooth. Transfer to a medium bowl
and serve with apple wedges or your choice of veggies.

Dinner

Sea Bass with Mango and Papaya Salsa

SERVES 6

Ingredients:

To marinate the fish:

¼ cup fresh lime juice (2 or 3 limes)

4 tablespoons plus 1 teaspoon extra-virgin olive oil

2 tablespoons finely chopped fresh oregano

½ teaspoon ground cumin

¼ teaspoon chili powder (optional)

¼ teaspoon sea salt

1½ pounds sea bass, red snapper, or rock fish fillets

2 limes, cut into wedges (optional)

For the mango salsa:

1 large, semiripe mango, peeled, cored, and cut into ½-inch pieces

1 large ripe papaya, peeled and cut into ½-inch pieces

½ red onion, finely diced

¼ to ½ serrano chile, finely diced (optional)

2 tablespoons finely chopped fresh cilantro

½ cup peeled and finely diced roasted red peppers (roast your own, for better flavor)

½ cup freshly squeezed lime juice

Sea salt to taste

Directions:

1. Marinate the fish: Whisk the lime juice, 3 tablespoons plus 2 teaspoons of the olive oil, the oregano, cumin, chili powder (if using), and salt together in a medium bowl. Add the fish fillets and turn to coat. Cover the bowl with plastic wrap and refrigerate for at least 1 hour or up to 3 hours.

2. Make the salsa: Toss the mango, papaya, and red onion in a bowl with the chile (if using), cilantro, roasted red peppers, and lime juice. Season with salt and refrigerate.

3. Heat a grill or a cast-iron grill pan to high heat. Carefully grease the grates or pan with the remaining 2 teaspoons olive oil. Remove the fish from the marinade and place on the grill. Cook for 4 to 5 minutes, until firm and no longer opaque. Remove bones if needed.

4. Top the sea bass with the salsa and fresh lime wedges.

Roasted Tomatoes

SERVES 4 AS A SIDE DISH

Ingredients:

4 cups cherry tomatoes
2 tablespoons extra-virgin olive oil
2 tablespoons balsamic vinegar
Sea salt to taste

Directions:

1. Preheat the oven to 350°F. Place the tomatoes in a 9 by 13-inch roasting pan, add the olive oil, and stir to coat. Roast for 45 minutes.
2. Remove from the oven, let cool slightly, then season with balsamic vinegar and sea salt.

Kale Caesar Salad with Quinoa

SERVES 4

Ingredients:

For the dressing:
1 head garlic
¼ cup extra-virgin olive oil
1 tablespoon Dijon mustard
1 tablespoon balsamic vinegar
⅛ teaspoon sea salt
½ can anchovies or sardines packed in olive oil, drained,
    1 tablespoon oil reserved for dressing (optional)

For the salad:
1 bunch lacinato/dinosaur kale, stems removed
1 fennel bulb
1 cup cooked quinoa
¼ cup toasted pine nuts

Directions:

1. Preheat the oven to 350°F. Slice a whole head of garlic in half crosswise and place inside a large piece of foil. Add a touch of extra-virgin olive oil to the inside, close the foil over the top to create an envelope, and roast for 45 minutes. Remove from the oven and cool. Squeeze the garlic cloves from the skins and chop.
2. While the garlic is cooking, slice the kale into thin ribbons. Cut the fennel bulb in half and thinly slice into half-moons using a mandoline.

3. In a large mixing bowl, whisk together the Dijon mustard, balsamic vinegar, and sea salt. Add the roasted garlic, mashing it with the back of a spoon to combine. Whisk in the olive oil and reserved sardine oil (if using) in a slow, steady stream until well blended.

4. Gently add the kale, cooked quinoa, and fennel to the dressing and toss well to coat. Add anchovies or sardines, if desired. Garnish with the toasted pine nuts.

Whole Lemon-Roasted Chicken

SERVES 6

Ingredients:

1 5- to 6-pound roasting chicken
¼ cup extra-virgin olive oil
1 teaspoon sea salt
1 lemon, thinly sliced into wheels
3 fresh thyme sprigs
3 fresh oregano sprigs
1 whole head garlic, unpeeled, broken into cloves

For the lemon-herb oil:
Juice of ½ lemon
2 tablespoons fresh thyme leaves, roughly chopped
2 tablespoons fresh oregano leaves, roughly chopped
2 tablespoons extra-virgin olive oil
1 teaspoon sea salt

Directions:

1. Preheat the oven to 400°F. Wash the chicken, remove the giblets, and pat completely dry with paper towels.
2. Lightly grease the bottom of a sturdy roasting pan with 2 tablespoons of the olive oil. Season the inside of the chicken with the sea salt and stuff the cavity with the lemon wheels, thyme and oregano sprigs, and garlic.
3. Using butcher's twine, truss the chicken breast-side-up, making sure to tuck in the wings and legs tightly. Place the chicken in the roasting pan and generously brush it with the remaining 2 tablespoons olive oil.

4. In a medium mixing bowl, whisk together all of the ingredients for the lemon-herb oil. Set aside.
5. Cover the chicken loosely with aluminum foil and roast for about 1½ hours. Remove the foil and roast for another 20 minutes. Remove the chicken from the oven and baste with the lemon-herb oil. Place back in the oven and continue cooking for about 10 minutes, uncovered, until golden brown and the internal temperature reaches 165°F.
6. Remove from the oven and let the chicken rest for 10 minutes. Serve with a squeeze of lemon and more fresh herbs on top.

Simple Herbed Salmon

SERVES 4

Ingredients:
4 6- to 8-ounce wild salmon fillets, skin on
Extra-virgin olive oil
Lemon wedge
Roasted tomatoes

For the marinade:
2 tablespoons extra-virgin olive oil
2 tablespoons fresh thyme leaves
2 tablespoons fresh oregano leaves
2 garlic cloves, finely minced
1 tablespoon fresh lemon juice, plus lemon wedges to serve
Sea salt to taste

Directions:

1. Preheat the oven to 350°F.
2. In a small mixing bowl, whisk together the ingredients for the marinade.
3. Add the salmon to the marinade, turning to coat both sides. Cover with plastic and refrigerate for 15 to 20 minutes.
4. Lightly grease a half sheet tray or 9 by 13-inch baking dish with olive oil and place the salmon fillets skin side down.
5. Bake for about 20 minutes, until the fish is opaque and firm to the touch. Remove from the oven and serve with a lemon wedge and a side of roasted tomatoes (page 128).

Smoky Sirloin Steak

SERVES 4

Ingredients:

1½ pounds top sirloin steak, trimmed
2 teaspoons extra-virgin olive oil

For the rub:
1 teaspoon smoked paprika
1 teaspoon garlic powder
1 teaspoon dried oregano
1 teaspoon sea salt

Directions:

1. To make the rub, stir the paprika, garlic powder, oregano, and sea salt together in a small bowl. Rub both sides of the steak with the spice mix. Place in a resealable plastic bag and refrigerate for at least 1 hour or overnight.
2. Remove the steak from the refrigerator and let it sit out at room temperature for 15 minutes. Carefully grease a grill or cast-iron grill pan with the olive oil and bring to medium-high heat. Place the steak on the grill or pan and cook for 3 or 4 minutes per side, until both sides are browned and nicely marked from the grill.
3. Transfer the steak to a cutting board and let it rest for 5 minutes before slicing against the grain into ½-inch-thick slices. Serve immediately.

Loaded Baked Potatoes

SERVES 4

Ingredients:

For the potatoes:
4 large russet potatoes
1 tablespoon extra-virgin olive oil
1 teaspoon sea salt

For the toppings:
1 tablespoon extra-virgin olive oil
½ yellow onion, roughly chopped
1 cup cremini or button mushrooms, thinly sliced
Chives, finely chopped (optional)
Sea salt

Directions:

1. Preheat the oven to 350°F. Line a baking sheet with aluminum foil and set aside. Pierce the potatoes several times with a fork. Place them in a bowl and toss with the olive oil and sea salt. Transfer the potatoes to the baking sheet and roast for approximately 1 hour, or until cooked through. Remove from the oven and set aside to cool slightly.
2. For the toppings, heat the olive oil in a medium skillet over medium heat. Add the onion and cook until soft and browned, about 10 minutes. Stir in the mushrooms and continue to cook until soft and fragrant, about 5 minutes more.
3. Cut a slit down the center of each potato and pinch the ends to open it up. Stuff each potato with 2 tablespoons of the mushroom mixture. To serve, sprinkle with chives, if desired, and additional sea salt to taste.

Bun-less Power Burger

MAKES 6 SLIDERS/SERVES 3

Ingredients:

For the patties:
2 tablespoons extra-virgin olive oil
1 yellow onion, finely diced
1 pound lean ground bison
2 tablespoons Worcestershire sauce
1 teaspoon sea salt
½ teaspoon freshly ground black pepper

Optional condiments:
12 large Bibb lettuce leaves
Dijon mustard
Organic ketchup
1 tomato, sliced
½ avocado, thinly sliced

Directions:

1. Heat 1 tablespoon of the olive oil in a large nonstick skillet over medium-high heat. Add the onion and cook for about 20 minutes, stirring occasionally, until golden brown.
2. Transfer the caramelized onions to a small bowl and set aside to cool. Clean the skillet for the bison patties.
3. Place the ground bison in a large mixing bowl. Add the Worcestershire sauce, salt, pepper, and the cooled caramelized onions. Mix well to combine. Form into patties 3½ inches in diameter and ½ inch thick.

4. Heat the remaining 1 tablespoon oil in the nonstick skillet over medium-high heat. Add the bison patties and cook until each side is browned and the burgers are cooked through, about 10 minutes total. Using a spatula, transfer the burgers to a large plate and set aside to rest for 5 minutes.

5. Place each burger on a Bibb lettuce leaf. Add a generous dollop of mustard and ketchup. Cover with a slice of tomato and avocado, top with another lettuce leaf, and serve.

Crispy Sweet Potato Fries

SERVES 6

Ingredients:

4 large sweet potatoes, scrubbed but unpeeled
2 teaspoons coconut oil, melted
½ teaspoon garlic powder
¾ teaspoon sea salt

Directions:

1. Preheat the oven to 450°F. Halve the sweet potatoes lengthwise and cut each half lengthwise into ½-inch wedges.

2. Place the sweet potatoes on a rimmed baking sheet. Drizzle the coconut oil over the potatoes. Add the garlic powder and ½ teaspoon of the salt and toss to coat. Roast the potatoes until golden brown and slightly crisp, 25 to 30 minutes. Sprinkle the potatoes with the remaining ¼ teaspoon salt. Serve alongside the Bun-less Power Burger (page 136).

Tuna Niçoise Salad

SERVES 4

Ingredients:

1 handful of green beans, trimmed
1 teaspoon sea salt
4 cups arugula
½ cup canned chickpeas, rinsed and drained
½ cup canned cannellini beans, rinsed and
  drained
2 plum tomatoes, thinly sliced lengthwise
¼ cup thinly sliced roasted red peppers
1 7-ounce can water-packed albacore tuna,
  drained
3 tablespoons balsamic vinegar
4 teaspoons Dijon mustard
1½ teaspoons honey
3 tablespoons extra-virgin olive oil

Directions:

1. Fill a medium saucepan with 1 inch of water. Place a steamer basket in the pot and bring the water to a simmer over high heat. Add the green beans, sprinkle with ¼ teaspoon of the sea salt, and reduce the heat to low. Cover and steam until tender, 5 to 6 minutes. Rinse the beans under cold water to stop the cooking. Drain and set aside.

2. Divide the arugula, chickpeas, cannellini beans, tomatoes, and roasted red peppers evenly among 4 shallow bowls.

Top each serving with one quarter of the tuna and arrange the green beans on top.

3. To make the vinaigrette, whisk the vinegar, mustard, honey, olive oil, and ½ teaspoon of the salt together in a small bowl. Drizzle the dressing over the salads and sprinkle each serving with some of the remaining salt.

Homemade Chicken Soup with Rice

SERVES 4

Ingredients:

1 head of roasted garlic
2 medium carrots, peeled and thinly sliced on the bias
2 celery stalks, thinly sliced on the bias
2 fresh thyme sprigs
2 tablespoons extra-virgin olive oil
2 quarts chicken stock, homemade or store-bought
1 cup brown rice
1 teaspoon sea salt, or to taste
2 cups shredded leftover chicken, white and dark meat

Directions:

1. To make roasted garlic: Cut a whole garlic bulb in half horizontally, rub with a touch of olive oil, and bake in a 350°F oven for about 1 hour, until soft. Set aside.

2. In a large stockpot over medium heat, sauté the carrots and celery with the thyme in the olive oil just until fragrant, about 5 minutes. Add the roasted garlic cloves. Gently pour the stock into the pot and simmer for about 15 minutes.

3. Add the rice and simmer over medium-low heat for 10 minutes.

4. Add sea salt to taste and the chicken. Simmer until the rice and carrots are tender, about 3 more minutes.

AFTERWORD

TALK A LOT in this book about change—how some simple adjustments to my diet made a huge difference in my career and my life. If you make positive changes that have half the impact on your life that mine had on me, I suspect you'll be very happy, and I'll be just as happy for you. But there's something else I need to tell you—a crucial point that I think gets lost in all the motivational white noise you hear out there.

When I'm standing on a tennis court, with another player—Nadal or Federer, for example—across the net, watching him bounce a ball and prepare to serve, I visualize that ball coming at me. The ball could take a dozen different trajectories, all to land in one small spot on the court to qualify as a nasty serve. Because I've seen those lines and angles thousands of times in real matches, I'm ready for them. I can react to them. I'm prepared.

That's what my endless practicing does for me. It prepares

me for whatever might happen on the court. It removes possibilities and replaces them with probabilities. The more you train, the more scenarios you experience and the fewer surprises you'll have. When, at the end of a long training session, my coach puts a small plastic water bottle on the court and makes me hit it with a full-on serve five more times before my day's work is done, knowing I have very little left in the tank and my focus is fraying . . . that's the stuff. That's what's going to separate me from another player four hours into a match.

Now, remember back to the beginning of this book, where I described what I felt like during tough matches, dating back just a couple of years ago? Remember how I fell apart, both mentally and physically, right around that three- or four-hour mark?

Physically, I couldn't compete. Mentally, I didn't feel like I belonged on the same court as the best players in the game. But then, lo and behold, I made some changes that transformed everything. Suddenly, that far into a match, I could *see*. I had the mental clarity to see those paths the serve could take, at 140 miles an hour, right to my racquet. I knew I could return anything and drop the ball wherever I needed to. I felt the energy crackling through my muscles. I had the explosive extra step I needed to beat the best in the world. To *be* the best in the world.

But understand, this wasn't magic: It wasn't the energy or the clarity or the renewed strength that allowed me to become the number one player in the world. It was my preparation. My training. The work ethic had always been there, starting with that six-year-old boy and his perfectly packed tennis bag. But suddenly there was an *X* factor, a change in my diet that allowed my body to perform the way it was meant to, without the allergies and the lethargy.

How does this apply to you?

It's simple. If you make these dietary changes, you may feel better. You may lose weight. You may look healthier. Your energy may spike. People may notice and compliment you. You may draw a few appreciative looks from attractive strangers.

Those are nice perks. But really, other than giving you a temporary ego boost and making you smile, what will any of that do for you?

Nothing.

Not a thing.

That's because weight loss and boundless energy aren't goals. And as much as you may think they're goals, I'd rather you see them as I do: gateways.

The real goal lies through the gateway.

That goal should be related to performance—in your career, in athletics, in relationships. Maybe you want a promotion, and your improved health allows you to perform at a higher level for a longer time each day. Maybe you want to start a dream business and you have the spark and drive you didn't have a year ago. Maybe you want to win a mixed-doubles tourney at the local court, or a basketball game, or maybe you want to finish a triathlon. Maybe you want to be closer to a spouse or partner, or find a *new* spouse or partner.

So here is my challenge to you, and the success secret I hope you understand: If you suddenly feel better, look better, and have the capacity to perform better . . . will you be prepared for it? Will you capitalize on it? Will you use it to rocket toward your goals?

I'll be honest—I never imagined that my new eating habits would make me feel so good. So capable. I always trained to be the best, but my body wouldn't let me see it through. Then suddenly, it did. And when the change happened and I felt amazing, I knew it would lead to *exactly* what I wanted to do: become number one in the world. Win, and keep winning.

Sure, I lost weight. Sure, I felt good. But that wasn't enough for me. I hope it's not enough for you.

Make the changes. Enjoy the process. But don't let the changes be your goal. Let them be your gateway to bigger, better goals.

Be ready.

ACKNOWLEDGMENTS

MUCH GRATITUDE IS DUE to my editor and collaborator, Stephen Perrine of Galvanized Brands, who helped distill my message into this useful and inspiring book.

Thanks also to Candice Kumai, who created many of the recipes you'll find in these pages, and who lives the same health-focused, gluten-free lifestyle that I do.

To the teams at Galvanized Brands and Random House, especially David Zinczenko, Libby Mcguire, Jennifer Tung, Nina Shield, Joe Heroun, Sara Vignieri, and John Mather, for their help with this project.

To Scott Waxman at Waxman Leavell Literary Agency and to Sandy Montag and Jill Driban at IMG for helping to make this deal a reality.

To the folks at American Media, Inc., and *Men's Fitness,* especially Andy Turnbull and Jane Seymour, and to Richard Phibbs, photographer, for making me look my best.

And to my fans, whose energy is critical to helping me stay focused and positive.

APPENDIX

THE GOOD FOOD GUIDE

"**H**OW DO YOU AVOID gluten? It's everywhere!"

That's the response I usually get when I tell people I'm gluten-free. They say the same thing about dairy and refined sugar.

And you know, they're right. When you eat foods that come in boxes and bags, it's almost impossible to avoid the additives you don't want. The key is to cut down on packaged and processed foods, and to check labels carefully.

But being surrounded by bad foods isn't the same as being forced to eat them. I'm able to avoid gluten, sugary foods, and dairy *easily*. It doesn't matter that they're "everywhere," because other foods—healthy, delicious, diverse foods—are everywhere, too.

That's the point of this chapter. If you want to try gluten-free, or sugar-free, or dairy-free—or all three—I understand if your first question is, "What's left for me to eat?"

The answer is . . . hundreds of foods in thousands of combinations. All of them healthy.

This appendix is proof that gluten-free is easier than you think. I've learned a lot about food in the past few years. Not just the foods that sabotage me, but the foods that help me win, day in, day out. I wanted to give you specific information about my favorite foods, what's in them, and why I like them (and yes, it's mostly because they taste great). And this isn't even a complete list!

PROTEIN

I like chicken, turkey, and all different kinds of fish. I eat one of these at least once or twice a day.

Eggs

I don't eat eggs often because I tend not to eat protein in the morning. But at the end of the day, they can make a very healthy, easy meal if you don't feel like cooking meat. Eggs are packed with nutrients (protein and selenium, for starters, at only 70–80 calories for a large egg), and they are incredibly versatile. Omelets alone make it easier to eat more vegetables.

Chicken (white meat)

A four-ounce boneless, skinless chicken breast has 24 grams of good, clean protein, B vitamins for energy, and about 125 calories. I always try to eat free-range, as those birds have more omega-3 fats than grain-fed chickens and flat-out taste better. When you buy chicken, watch out for added salt. Some poultry producers inject solutions into chicken breasts to make them juicier and more flavorful. A four-ounce breast typically has 50 to 70 milligrams of sodium; a plumped-up piece can push 500 mg. *Read the label.*

Turkey (white meat)

Turkey breast is nutritionally similar to chicken breast—28 grams of protein with 125 calories in four ounces, and lots of B vitamins.

Turkey (ground)

Just be sure to read the label and go for white meat. Most ground turkey is a combination of light and dark, which raises your calorie intake and lowers your protein content per four-ounce serving.

Beef

I don't go crazy with red meat because to me it's very heavy, but I enjoy it occasionally. Beef is loaded with protein, obviously, but also with monounsaturated fats, zinc, B vitamins, and iron. Grass-fed beef, if it's available, has a much higher ratio of omega-3 fats to omega-6 fats (about 1:3, versus 1:20 in corn-fed beef). High levels of omega-6 fats cause inflammation, which no one needs.

Oh, and one other thing to watch out for: I typically eat about a four-ounce serving of beef as a meal, which gives me about 250 calories. If you order steak in a restaurant, understand that your serving will be much bigger than four ounces. I've seen ridiculous forty-eight-ounce steaks on menus—that's four pounds! Everyone is different, but I know that if I eat anything more than an eight-ounce steak, I'll feel lousy for hours.

Wild Alaskan Salmon (sockeye)

Avoid farmed (or "Atlantic") salmon every time. It's far lower in nutrients than wild and is even fed artificial pigments to make its meat a more appealing shade of pinkish-orange. Ugh. But a nice piece of salmon is amazing for you: lots of B vitamins and selenium, about 24 grams of protein and 175 calories in a four-ounce serving. And it's full of heart-healthy fats, which raise good HDL cholesterol levels.

Yellowfin Tuna and other fish

Tuna packs a higher protein dose per calories than most fish—28 grams for just 125 calories—and it's high in omega-3s. When you're shopping at the fish counter, know that tuna is never naturally brown. It should be bright red. Other healthy fish: sardines, mackerel, rainbow trout, arctic char.

Shellfish

Shrimp, lobster, and clams are all high in protein and low in calories. Just don't dip them in butter.

VEGETABLES

Yes, they're the primary natural source of virtually every nutrient a human can need: vitamins, minerals, fiber, and antioxidants. But not all vegetables are created equal. Some—particularly root vegetables and winter vegetables—are heavy in starch and carbohydrates, and since I try to eat the majority of my carbohydrates during the day, for maximum energy, I typically avoid these at dinner, when I am focusing on protein. But leafy and stalk vegetables are what I call "neutral." They aren't high in carbs, so I eat them at any time of day, and with every meal.

Neutral vegetables

These all tend to be high in fiber and vitamins A, B, C, and K, and low in calories, so eat them any time: asparagus, artichokes, Brussels sprouts, cabbage, broccoli, cauliflower, bok choy, broccoli rabe, mustard greens, Swiss chard, spinach, dandelion, kale, watercress, arugula, summer squash, zucchini, red bell peppers (which are much more nutritious than green ones), and green-leaf, red-leaf, and romaine lettuce.

High-carb vegetables

These I eat only during the day, when I'm seeking energy. While they are all packed with fiber and vitamins, especially vitamin A, they are too carbohydrate-rich for my evening meals: corn, potatoes, onions, sweet potatoes, parsnips, carrots, beets, peas, turnips, winter squash (like acorn and butternut), and pumpkin.

Olives

They're a wonderful anti-inflammatory food and add a punch of flavor to a salad.

BEANS AND LEGUMES

A warning: Too many can make your digestion more musical than you'd like. And try to avoid canned beans, because they are high in sodium. Buy them dry and soak them overnight: black beans, edamame, chickpeas (hummus), fava beans, green beans, peas, lentils, navy beans, black-eyed peas, kidney beans, cannellini beans, and lima beans.

FRUITS

Your body needs the healthy sugar—fructose—that comes from fruits. I eat a lot of fruit during the day for energy, but seldom at night; again, in the evening, I'm telling my body to process protein, and I don't want to confuse it with too many carbohydrate calories.

High-sugar fruits

These taste delicious and are one of the most nutritionally dense foods available. Basically, the idea of an "apple a day" is spot-on, assuming you watch your sugar the rest of the day. High-sugar fruits include apples, pears, grapes, cherries, peaches, nectarines, apricots, plums, strawberries, raspberries, blackberries, and blueberries. One thing you'll notice about these is that they all have edible skins. That makes them very high in pesticides, so I try to eat organic versions of these fruits whenever possible.

Bananas, figs, and papaya

All are high in nutrients, and bananas and figs are among the best sources of potassium, which helps prevent heart disease and high blood pressure. But they are also very high in sugar, so eat them in moderation.

Citrus and other high-acid fruits

Because you don't typically eat the skins, there's no need to buy organic oranges, grapefruits, lemons, limes, pineapples, mangos, guavas, passion fruit, kiwis, and pomegranates. Be aware that all of these are high in nutrients (especially vitamin C) *and* calories. And skip juices—orange juice has many more calories than an orange, and none of the fiber.

Dried fruit

I'm very careful about dried fruit: raisins, dried apricots, dates, and prunes. On one hand, they're loaded with nutrition. But they also deliver a big dose of sugar. Take them in moderation and use them for portable energy when you're active.

Tomatoes

Yes, tomatoes are fruits. I have a mild sensitivity to them, but I still enjoy them occasionally, as long as they are fresh and not processed (I eat only tomato sauce made from fresh tomatoes, for example). Lycopene, the phytochemical that makes tomatoes red, helps eliminate skin-aging free radicals caused by ultraviolet rays.

Avocado

Here's another fruit usually listed in the vegetable section. Avocadoes may be my favorite food. Big flavor, big fiber, big nutrition. And you can do so much with a fresh avocado. It is very high in healthy, monounsaturated fats.

WHEAT-ALTERNATIVE GRAINS

Many supermarkets now have gluten-free sections, and of course, you can always order dried pastas, crackers, and other products over the Internet. There are some very good wheat-alternative grains available these days. If you've never tried them, I suggest seeking them out and experimenting. I most often go with quinoa, buckwheat, brown rice, and oats. Quinoa and buckwheat make a tasty gluten-free pasta.

Quinoa

The South American grain quinoa (KEEN-wah) has about twice as much fiber and protein as brown rice, and its protein consists of a complete set of branch chain and essential amino acids, so it helps build muscle better than other grains. All that protein and fiber—in conjunction with a handful of healthy fats and a comparatively small dose of carbohydrates—lower the insulin response. Quinoa also tastes great and cooks up in 15 minutes.

Oats (instant, old-fashioned, and steel-cut)

Instant (and one-minute) oatmeal is basically rolled oats cut up to cook faster. Old-fashioned oatmeal consists of groats (the actual grains) rolled into flakes; it takes about five minutes to cook. Steel-cut is made of groats that are cut up but not rolled; it takes a half hour to cook. Oats are one of the easiest ways to get more fiber into your diet and contain lots of protein, too. I like steel-cut because the pure grain doesn't raise your blood sugar as much as the more processed varieties. Watch out for supermarket brands that add tons of sugar. Best to have it plain with some fruit or nuts.

Brown Rice

Plain brown rice is what I call a fallback food. There are other grains that I like better for nutrition and taste, but brown rice is available everywhere and works when other favorites (like quinoa or gluten-free pasta) aren't available. It delivers a strong dose of minerals and fiber and is a good vehicle for other foods (and I'm sure I don't have to tell you to sub it in for white rice, right?).

Buckwheat

I love buckwheat pasta. And buckwheat itself is strong stuff. One ounce has 3 grams of fiber and 4 grams of protein, plus minerals such as copper, magnesium, and manganese. A lot of these gluten-free grains have become staples in my diet, with buckwheat one of the biggest.

Millet

Millet is a gluten-free grain from Asia that's nutritionally comparable to wheat: An ounce has 2 grams of fiber, 3 grams of protein, plus B vitamins, calcium, and iron. I've seen millet used as a wheat substitute in oatmeal muffins, cereal, and even stuffed tomatoes.

Muesli

Muesli, a combination of rolled oats, dried fruits, and nuts, originally came from Switzerland. I use it almost every day as an ingredient in my Power Bowl. A cup pushes 300 calories, but that's the point: It's a foundation of my morning diet. It has a huge payoff with fiber and protein, plus vitamins B and E, iron, and more.

Shirataki

This isn't a grain, but it seems to fit here. Shirataki is a low- or no-carb noodle from Asia that's translucent and made from the root of the Asian konjac yam. Researchers in Thailand found that just 1 gram has the power to significantly slow the absorption of sugar into your bloodstream. They have no real flavor, but they will soak up the flavor of whatever food they're prepared with.

Amaranth

Amaranth is one of the most powerful grains, nutrition-wise. It's gluten-free, for one, and higher in fiber and protein than wheat and brown rice. It's loaded with vitamins and has been shown in studies to help lower blood pressure and cholesterol. Also, it's a muscle builder, since it's one of the few grains that contain "complete" proteins, i.e., all eight essential amino acids.

Teff

Teff comes from Ethiopia. There are brown and ivory varieties, and I find the brown to be more flavorful—both sweet and nutty. A cup has 6 grams of fiber and 10 grams of protein, as well as plenty of minerals. It's easy to prepare, too: Just throw a cup in with 3 cups of boiling water and simmer for about 20 minutes. Play with your favorite spices for taste—teff works with just about anything.

Spaghetti squash

A vegetable, actually, but if you cut open a spaghetti squash, its insides look like spaghetti and can even be used as a gluten-free pasta alternative. Use it as a vehicle for other foods, because this squash isn't that high in nutrition.

NUTS AND SEEDS

These help keep me fueled and full as my training day goes on. I have raw, not roasted, whenever possible. It's easy to control the amount you eat (a handful is a great snack), so they deliver protein without weighing you down, and deliver fiber and monounsaturated fats, too. Add almonds, pistachios, cashews, walnuts, pecans, Brazil nuts, macadamia nuts, peanuts, flaxseed, sunflower seeds, pumpkin seeds, sesame seeds, hemp seeds, or chia seeds to salads, cereals, or even smoothies.

HEALTHY OILS (FATS)

Without fat, your body can't absorb most vitamins. I use oils sparingly. Here are the ones I do eat.

Olive Oil
The go-to oil. By now you must know about the healthy fats in olive oil. Extra-virgin has a robust flavor and is most expensive, so people generally use it for salad dressings, vegetables, and dipping (though everyone loves bread dipped in olive oil, I've had to give that up). Lighter olive oil is good for cooking.

Canola Oil
Great for frying and sautéing if olive oil isn't an option. Canola oil can withstand relatively high heat, and its neutral flavor won't dominate a recipe. Just be careful: Don't confuse canola with generic "vegetable oil," which is cheaper and

usually made from soybean or corn oil. Those oils have high levels of omega-6 fatty acids. These polyunsaturated fats aren't bad when they're balanced with plenty of omega-3 fatty acids, like the ones found in fish—and canola oil. Basically, omega-6s can cause inflammation in your body, and omega-3s have anti-inflammatory properties, so you want to balance them out as much as possible.

Coconut oil

Some people are scared off by the saturated fat in coconut oil, thinking that it raises cholesterol. It does, but the lauric acid in the oil has been shown to raise HDL (good cholesterol). On top of that, studies have shown coconut oil to be an immune-system booster that can also help the body use insulin more effectively. The "oil" doesn't look like regular oils in that it comes as a solid, like shortening (without the trans fats). I've seen people drop a teaspoon in coffee and it also works well in smoothies and as a shortening substitute in baking.

Flaxseed oil

Flaxseed oil is high in alpha-linolenic acid, which is an anti-inflammatory and can help lower your cholesterol. I like it because it's a healthier oil than most out there and our bodies can't produce the essential fatty acids in the oil by themselves.

Nut butters

Peanut butter is very healthy, as long as it has only one ingredient: peanuts. So check the label to make sure there's no added sugar, salt, or palm oil. Other nut butters, particularly almond butter, are even healthier choices.

Avocado, walnut, and hazelnut oils

Perfect for salad dressings or mixing into foods, they add great flavor and a hit of monounsaturated fats.

DAIRY SUBSTITUTES

Be wary of "non-dairy creamers" and other chemical concoctions. They're often high in sugar and unhealthy fats. If you're going to cut out dairy, look for these alternatives to milk, yogurt, and ice cream: almond milk, coconut milk, rice milk, hazelnut milk. I generally avoid soy milk because of its high concentration of soy isolates, which have estrogenic properties—in other words, it's bad for your muscles and can lead to fat storage.

ABOUT THE AUTHOR

Novak Djokovic is a Serbian tennis player who is ranked World No. 1 by the Association of Tennis Professionals. He is widely considered to be one of the greatest tennis players of all time.

novakdjokovic.com